'A book that's likely to threaten all the doctor-knows-best volumes that litter the pregnancy book shelves, *Alternative Therapies for Pregnancy and Birth* gathers together into one outstanding, easy-to-navigate volume all the information you need. This essential pregnancy bible for the holistic mother-to-be takes a deeper view of the entire experience, with excellent advice about spiritual matters and the thorny issue of how baby-makes-three changes a relationship. Pat Thomas is fast becoming the Miriam Stoppard of natural pregnancy.'

Lynne McTaggart, editor of *What Doctors Don't Tell You* and *Natural Parent*

'Pat Thomas reminds us that pregnancy is a natural event and not an illness and gives women practical advice to take control of both their pregnancy and childbirth.'

Dr Marilyn Glenville PhD, author of *Natural Solutions to Infertility*

'This is a thorough and well-researched book which is very comprehensive in its scope. Pat Thomas questions complementary therapies as much as she does conventional treatment. You can be sure that the advice contained in *Alternative Therapies for Pregnancy and Birth* is very sound. This is an invaluable resource which women seeking alternative forms of care in pregnancy and empowerment for birth can rely on.'

Janet Balaskas, Founder of the Active Birth Centre and author of *New Natural Pregnancy*

'If you are the kind of woman who believes that your body is your responsibility and birth is not a medical event to be endured, this is for you. Pat Thomas's thoughtful and extensive exploration of alternative therapies should be read by every woman who takes responsibility for her own, and her baby's health.'

Beverley Beech, Chair for the Association for Improvements in the Maternity Services (AIMS)

'Read and read again the central paragraph of Pat's book: "Everything in moderation – even awareness." There is food for thought in every single sentence … including the reference to the hypnotic effect of the click clack of knitting needles in a quiet room. It makes me think of the forgotten art of midwifery.'

Michael Odent, Primal Health Research Centre

Alternative Therapies for Pregnancy and Birth

Pat Thomas

vega

A catalogue record for this book is available
from the British Library.

ISBN UK 1-84333-007-5
ISBN US 1-84333-713-4
Printed in Great Britain by
Creative Print and Design Group, Wales.

© Vega 2001

A member of the Chrysalis Group plc

Published in 2001 by
Vega
64 Blenheim Court
Brewery Road
London N7 9NY

Visit our website at
www.chrysalisbooks.co.uk

Note from the publisher.
Any information given in this book is not intended
to be taken as a replacement for medical advice.
The reader is strongly urged to consult a qualified
medical practitioner or suitable therapist before
trying any of the treatments mentioned

CONTENTS

This book is dedicated, with love, to my late mother –

who never understood there was an alternative.

ACKNOWLEDGEMENTS

From the very beginning, the scope of this book was enormous. I am therefore grateful to those people who helped me keep my perspective during its compilation, writing and editing.

I am indebted to Alice Charlwood and Beverley Beech for their perceptive comments on the early drafts; and to Joanna Goldberg for casting a sub-editor's eye over the text. I am especially grateful to Jeremy Gilbey for his comments on osteopathy and chiropractic, to Stephen Terrass for his insight into nutritional therapy, and to Nadine Edwards and Andrea McLaughlin for their input in the yoga and Alexander Technique chapter.

Thanks to my agent Laura Longrigg for her continuing guiding hand.

Finally, many people in my life showed extraordinary patience with me while I sifted (not always good-naturedly) through the mountains of papers, journals and books that formed the background to this work: my son Alexander, his father Jonathan, and everyone at AIMS and the Wallace Press. Bless you.

MOVING FORWARD

Pregnancy is a time of choices. It is a life event in which a woman is and must be an active participant.

Often, the way a woman is treated by some of the health professionals she may encounter during pregnancy suggests that her role is merely that of a passive patient – waiting for appointments and test results, lying on her back for examinations and delivery. But there comes a day in every pregnancy when the truth dawns. From the moment of conception, a mother is making choices and decisions for herself and her baby – nutritionally, aesthetically, physically, emotionally, educationally and psychologically. While it may seem that there are already too many options for pregnant women, appearances can be deceptive. What pregnant woman are offered from mainstream medicine can be likened to the choices on a menu. In other words, women are obliged, or so it seems, to select only what a particular hospital or clinic wishes to offer.

Some women, understandably, feel overwhelmed by the responsibility of making choices at this time. Yet even opting out and simply going along with what is on offer is a choice which, along with all the others a woman makes about her pregnancy care, may directly affect the outcome of her pregnancy. It is a well-kept secret that empowering women with information and encouraging them to make independent choices about their maternity care results in better outcomes – fewer sick or dead babies and mothers – irrespective of the choices they make.

To help ease this burden, many women turn for help to antenatal teachers, midwives and doctors (and even authors). Today's professionals and experts have taken the place of the extended family. In more traditional cultures, a pregnant woman would be surrounded by grandmothers, mothers, sisters, aunts, nieces and female friends, who would be there to support and advise. But the isolation of the modern family means that women must often go outside their usual social and familial group for help and advice. The problems of seeking information this way are manifold.

In seeking help from an obstetrician, a woman may be largely unaware that obstetrics is a speciality dealing with *complicated* or *high-risk* pregnancies. The obstetrician's view will be heavily weighted towards medical care, not because medical care is best for all pregnant women, but because it is what the obstetrician knows best.

General practitioners are hard workers but, by and large, they do not have the time to be deep thinkers. They are not usually well informed about healthcare alternatives and are likely to underestimate the importance of basics such as nutrition, because medical training pays minimal lip-service to such matters. Medical training also frowns upon independent thought. It avoids discussions about emotion, philosophy, psychology and personal value systems because these blur the edges of diagnosis, making the process much harder and more time-consuming. Our family doctors are trained in disease management, not health promotion, and for this reason (and the fact that the majority of GPs have never delivered a baby or seen a normal birth) they are not always the best choice for information about pregnancy – which is, after all, a state of health.

Midwives are the only practitioners who are trained to facilitate normal birth, but across the world the profession of midwifery is being hounded into extinction. If this sounds overly dramatic, consider the editorial in the respected medical journal *The Lancet* in 1998 – which described the destruction of midwifery as a 'global witch hunt'.

Those who practise privately – known as independent midwives – are now the only midwives who are free to use the full range of their skills. Yet their numbers are dwindling drastically all over the world. Today, many hospital-based midwives are not much more than low-status lackeys and clerks, carrying out the consultant's instructions and upholding the policies of the local health authority. While information from your midwife is likely to be more weighted towards health promotion and the goal of a normal birth, this will not always be the case.

Antenatal teachers also vary in their approaches to birth and the information they provide. Some exist mainly to explain the hospital routine to new mothers, while others actively promote the idea of natural birth. While the latter may seem a better choice, those who champion 'natural birth' often omit to tell women that such a thing is nearly impossible within a hospital setting. Few are skilled in helping the woman who, in spite of the odds, wishes to pursue a natural birth *and* a hospital birth, to negotiate her needs effectively within a bureaucratic system. You may have to look hard to find someone who is knowledgeable and effective and who understands the primary function of the childbirth educator: the passing on of accurate information and practical skills to prospective parents.

Readers of this and other books, be aware! Authors, too, have taken the place of family members. Buying books about pregnancy has become yet another way of seeking support. That pile of baby books by the bed, on the coffee table or in the bathroom is the means by which many women attempt to decode, more or less independently, the mystery of pregnancy and birth and make sense of their place in it all. It is becoming increasingly important for women to learn to distinguish between those which are simply regurgitating common 'policy' and those which aim to provide deeper insight, inspiration and a context for the experience of being pregnant and giving birth.

PART I
ON THE THRESHOLD

CHAPTER 1

EXPECTING MORE

There has never been a time in history when simply being pregnant and giving birth has seemed so complicated. This is because there has never been a time in history when being a woman has seemed so complicated. Whatever gains we imagine we have made in work, in relationships and in the wider culture, the struggle to find a positive definition of what it is to be a woman, particularly with regard to our reproductive lives, is as intense as ever. Nowhere is that struggle felt as keenly as in the arena of pregnancy and birth.

Being pregnant and giving birth involve more than simply growing and expelling a live baby. The whole process, when entered into positively and openly, can play a valuable part in reconnecting us with some of the positive aspects of being a woman. It can help us to listen to our bodies and let our lives be informed by them. It can enrich our lives with a sense of connection, where communication can happen in silence or through physical contact. It compels us to defocus and let go; to live not so much for the end-goal, but for the experience. It teaches us the value of sitting still and waiting in a world where everything needs to be done yesterday. These are just some elements of the 'feminine' which continue to be eroded in our culture.

In truth, many women who allow themselves to be full participants in the experience of pregnancy and birth rarely express their feelings in such lofty terms; usually they just say it 'feels right'.

This book is written from the point of view that there are legitimate alternatives to the common experience of pregnancy and birth which so many women find anxiety-provoking and mechanistic. Primarily, it is a book about healthcare alternatives, but within that context it is also a book about physiological, emotional and psychological alternatives. Using alternative healthcare provides an opportunity to reframe our thinking about a whole range of issues which arise for women during pregnancy and birth. It provides a way to step, fully supported, outside a system of lowest-common-denominator care into a world where pregnancy is not treated as an illness and where the pregnant woman is defined as the primary expert on her own body and her baby.

The information here isn't just distilled from research and science but from a variety of sources. Where possible, it comes from the experience of mothers themselves. It presents pregnancy and birth in the context of a life event, not a medical one. If you are having your first child, it can be very difficult to envisage any way to proceed other than the way your doctor advises. It may not occur to you that a doctor's advice is sometimes based on habit rather than an interest in your individual needs or even the most current medical evidence. Often it takes tremendous courage for first-time mothers to question, criticize and even reject those aspects of conventional care which they feel uncomfortable with. Intuitions and nagging doubts – and every woman has them – tend to be reduced to a small voice, easily drowned out by the unceasing noise of modern antenatal care.

Women who have already had babies, on the other hand, especially those who have been able to process the experience sensitively and intelligently, possess a special knowledge which can and should be used to support less experienced women in their choices. These are the women who don't just ask for more choices; they often insist on them and use them to good effect. This is in part because they have learned that the experience of pregnancy and birth will stay with them for ever. Some carry bitter memories of inadequate or inappropriate care during a first pregnancy and are not keen to experience the same thing again. Others simply feel that they would like to do it differently this time around and be more in control.

> '*Pay* attention to
> *the pregnant woman!*
> *There is no one as*
> *important as she.*'
> CHAGGA SAYING, UGANDA

It is shocking to find out that the majority of unnecessary interventions, both antenatally and in labour, are carried out on first-time mothers. There is no biological reason for this. There is little physiological difference between the body of a woman who has had children and that of a woman who has not. Both are physically capable of giving birth with a minimum of intervention. What is different is the mind, the emotions and the level of confidence. First-timers tend to be more compliant patients, whereas second-timers are more inclined to dictate their own terms. If you are a first-timer you could learn a great deal from those who have learned to expect more – of themselves and of those around them.

Although birth is an intensely personal experience, it has another side as well. Being pregnant expands your knowledge of the world, how it works and who is perceived to be in control. This is why it is sometimes experienced as a political, as well as a personal, event. Although pregnancy is an exclusively female experience, it is managed almost exclusively by men (and occasionally by women inspired by macho ideology). Through medical management, women are told what to expect and what action they should take (i.e. tests, drugs or surgery). To enter pregnancy as a fully conscious woman is to accept the challenge to stop 'taking it like a man' and respond instead from your own genuine self. Those who take up the challenge often experience a deep radicalization of their world views.

WHAT'S WRONG WITH CONVENTIONAL CARE?

Pregnancy can be a surprisingly powerful time in a woman's life. Unfortunately, too many women experience it from a position of utter powerlessness, anxiety and frustration. In the eyes of conventional medicine, pregnancy has become a disorder which women fall victim to and which only doctors can cure, increasingly by removing the baby in the same manner as they would any other 'growth'.

Too often we choose to associate pregnancy with illness and the need for medical care. We accept the negative images of pregnant women – sickly, easily confused, hormonally challenged – in much the same way that we choose to associate breastfeeding women with 'cows' and not more powerful and inspiring mammals such as lionesses, gazelles or even dolphins.

This is one of the main problems with the way Western medics manage pregnancy and birth – it can be so undermining. It can reinforce some widespread and powerful insecurities which women have about their bodies, heightening a sense of fear, bewilderment and helplessness rather than promoting skill, competence and confidence. Then (in the great tradition of all romantic fictions), when the woman's confidence in herself and her baby has all but disappeared, conventional medicine offers a hero, in the form of the doctor, who will save the bewildered female from her terrible ordeal. The question remains: do women really need to be saved from pregnancy and birth?

Within the system of medical care doctors and midwives also, ironically, look to others to save them from their bewilderment and lack of insight. These 'others' are machines and lab tests. This is another disturbing aspect of conventional 'care', which brings with it a loss of practical, clinical skills among healthcare professionals and the tendency to reduce mothers to nothing more than the sum total of their test results and 'risk' factors.

While tests and technology can be useful, and for some reassuring, in recent years antenatal testing has become aggrandized within our hospitals and clinics. So much so that few practitioners now feel confident to pronounce a woman well and her baby healthy without a stack of test results in front of them. Often, however, this blind faith in technology is not justified. An alarmingly large proportion of commonly used procedures have been shown to be of no benefit – in other words they do not improve the outcome of the pregnancy – for either mother or baby. Some may even do harm.

One example of such a technology is repeated exposure to ultrasound. Heaven help the woman who rejects the opportunity to have a scan. She will be asked, sometimes repeatedly, to justify such a bizarre decision and may be accused of wantonly putting her baby in

In American Indian culture, the Shaman was aware that any procedure or remedy given to the patient would change them in some profound way. The Shaman would always ask the spirits (and the patient) for permission to change the course of an individual's life before performing any procedure intended to help or heal. How different things might be if our modern doctors did this before performing an ultrasound scan, an episiotomy or a caesarean!

danger. Yet, such a woman may have sound reasons for declining the opportunity (*see* the chart in chapter 2, pages 36–7). For all its day-to-day use, and the joy which some parents experience in seeing their baby for the first time, mothers are not told that ultrasound is still wholly unevaluated with regard to its long-term safety.

Many women dislike hearing this, especially since most will have at least two scans during pregnancy and will be exposed to repeated doses of ultrasound whenever the fetal heart monitor is used. Yet, the energy output of ultrasound machines is becoming increasingly high and studies exist which suggest a link between as few as two or three antenatal scans and subtle brain damage as well as arrested cell development in the developing fetus. When it comes to ultrasound we tend to confuse value with evaluation. No evaluation has taken place to help us predict which babies are most at risk of being damaged by ultrasound. However, increasing amounts of research are showing that repeated scans are no better than a single scan for improving birth outcomes and that scans are producing more *false positives* – diagnoses of abnormality where there is none, leading to unnecessary terminations of wanted pregnancies – and *false negatives* – missing abnormalities and providing false reassurance for anxious couples. The woman who rejects the scan may simply feel that she does not wish to take part in what appears to be a medical version of Russian Roulette.

It is interesting to reflect upon how women who accept repeated scanning during pregnancy would respond if they were asked to justify their actions in the same way.

There are other commonly used procedures which research has found make little difference to influencing outcomes, and indeed can make things considerably worse. These include continuous electronic fetal monitoring during labour which has been shown to increase the risk of unnecessary caesarean operations through the false diagnosis of fetal distress; artificial rupture of the membranes (breaking the waters in early labour), shown to increase the risk of infection and cord prolapse; caesarean operations – increasing the risk of infection, haemorrhage and even death due to anaesthetic complications, as well as reducing future fertility; and syntocinon – a synthetic hormone used to induce labour, now associated with increased risk of haemorrhage and cerebral palsy, as well as higher levels of pain and fetal distress during labour.

In some hospitals, more than 70 per cent of women commonly receive these procedures (often one on top of the other). And although women have the right to refuse any or all of these interventions at any time, why would they when everything they have gleaned from the hospital 'menu' indicates that these things are safe and desirable? What is more, these procedures are, from a medical standpoint, a necessary part of 'doing birth right'. Some women, it must be said, also equate the amount of 'stuff' done to them with good, responsible care and the acceptance of this 'stuff' with being a good, responsible parent. In so doing they help to perpetuate the idea that interference is only intervention and that control is, in reality, care.

WHY ALTERNATIVE MEDICINE?

Most illnesses are never reported to the family doctor. This is partly because women provide a vast amount of family healthcare within the community. Women bandage knees, cool fevers, ease stomach upsets, earaches and headaches and advise on everything from acne to ingrown toenails to piles. Women are also the ones most likely to consider self-help options for themselves. Often, this care involves the use of over-the-counter medicines. However, once a woman is pregnant, she is unlikely to want to use any medicine which could potentially harm her baby. For this reason, pregnancy is the time when many women investigate alternative remedies for the first time.

Alternative medicine can no longer be considered a fringe interest. Studies in both the UK and the US show that more than 40 per cent of healthcare consumers will turn to alternative medicine before they will go to a conventional doctor. Visits to alternative practitioners are up by nearly 50 per cent across the Western world.

Alternative therapies are particularly appropriate during pregnancy since they take an holistic view of health care. In other words, they place no boundaries between physical, emotional and mental well-being. In pregnancy these boundaries also begin to disappear; how a woman's body is developing has a direct effect on how she thinks and feels and

Women have always shown courage in taking difficult decisions with regard to their health, even to the point of performing caesareans on themselves. The earliest known case was recorded in 1769 in the West Indies and the last recorded case was in Italy in 1886. It sounds risky, but interestingly, in 1944, an American medical historian, R.P. Harris, recorded a 66 per cent survival and recovery rate for women performing the operation on themselves, but only a 37.5 per cent rate for those operated on by American physicians (and 14 per cent for their British counterparts). There were many reasons for the discrepancy. One was that women carrying out the operation on themselves were more likely to be using clean kitchen implements, whereas in the hospitals of the day surgeons rarely washed their equipment from one patient to another.

vice versa. In alternative medicine there is a broader definition of good health. It encompasses more than the mere absence of symptoms, because even in the absence of symptoms, a patient's essential vitality and ability to resist illness may be low. An alternative therapist may be able to discern this and work with the patient to help strengthen and maintain a healthy immune system. This is an especially important consideration during pregnancy, when all the major body systems come under unaccustomed stress.

Also, in holistic healthcare no aspect of the self is too trivial; posture, lifestyle, beliefs and values, energy and work and their impact on the total picture of a person's health are all relevant.

Because of this, there is a certain amount of personal responsibility put upon the individual who seeks alternative forms of care. You must do what you can to help yourself, whether it means changing your diet, taking the idea of relaxation seriously and integrating it into your life, or taking more exercise. It may also encompass more difficult tasks such as facing up to uncomfortable aspects of your past, examining your own beliefs and behaviour and looking objectively at some of your relationships and priorities. A good alternative therapist will usually have something to say about all these aspects of your life and may be able to refer you, should you wish, to others who can be of assistance.

Readers may be wondering at this point about the use of the term 'alternative' as opposed to complementary. The choice is deliberate. The goals of most holistic therapies are often quite different from those of conventional medicine and the use of the word alternative is informed by a bigger picture, not just of general healthcare, but of pregnancy and birth.

Many of the aims of holistic healthcare are diametrically opposed to those of conventional medicine. For instance, alternative medicine is aimed at self-healing and prevention rather than reacting to and suppressing symptoms as they arise. The idea of partnership with the therapist is also in opposition to the dominant-subordinate relationships which many doctors and patients have. Alternative medicine believes in the innate ability of the body to heal itself, conventional medicine believes that only medicine or surgery can cure.

Perhaps most importantly to the pregnant woman, the therapies, when practised competently by her and/or her chosen practitioner, are generally safe and remedies such as herbs and homeopathy are for the most part harmless and non-toxic. While any medicine, even the natural ones, can potentially produce adverse effects, these are very rare when compared to those of conventional medicine.

In contrast to conventional medicine, which is most at home treating acute diseases, alternative medicine has much to offer those who suffer from chronic complaints. And because many alternative therapies can be practised at home, they also place healthcare squarely in the context of the community rather than in isolated bureaucratic centres. These distinctions will perhaps blur over time, but for now the most fundamental principles of holistic healing are so different from those of conventional medicine that they can only be regarded as an 'alternative'.

By using alternative therapies, many women are finding a way to take back control of their own pregnancies and keep the system, which encourages women to switch off and leave it all to the 'experts', at bay. Indeed, the self-help element of many alternative therapies emphasizes the woman's role as her own expert, and this is one of the driving ideas behind this book.

You don't need a PhD, or a degree of any kind, to understand your body – you live in it. Every woman, even if she is expecting her first child, is a potential expert on pregnancy and birth. Often all that is lacking is appropriate information and support. The holistic philosophy of many alternative systems of healthcare puts the woman exactly where she should be – at the centre of her own experience. It can instil a sense of confidence and calm and provide an important counterbalance to the impersonal procedures and panicked search for pathology that characterizes many hospitals and antenatal clinics.

Nevertheless, opting out of conventional care can sometimes prove difficult and emotionally challenging. Many women who choose to pursue alternative forms of care find that they are not supported by their caregivers or their families, who fear that in rejecting some or all aspects of conventional care they are endangering themselves and their child. Such fear is born of ignorance, and this book goes some way towards addressing such ignorance. The practicalities of refusing multiple scans, opting for a vaginal breech birth or booking a home or water birth, however, are complex and beyond the scope of this book. Good evidence-based information on this subject, including my own *Every Woman's Birth Rights* (*see* the Bibliography, page 292, for more suggestions), is plentiful, and women should exercise their right to seek support and information which can help them arrange an antenatal and birth experience with which they feel comfortable.

As you begin to consider your alternatives in healthcare during pregnancy and in labour, and incorporate these into your birth plan (*see* appendix 1, page 287), try not to think in terms of substituting one pill or procedure for another. Many of the most effective strategies in maternity care are 'non-active'. They involve trust, caring, affection, instinct and emotional support. This is good advice, because while you are many times less likely to experience an adverse reaction to alternative remedies, it is not unheard of. For instance, herbal medicine is the closest thing the alternative world has to conventional drugs. Many herbs provide the blueprint for today's conventional medicines. Used wisely, herbs can provide a safe alternative to conventional drugs. Used unwisely, or without respect, they can also produce unwanted side-effects.

For this reason, it is advisable to establish the idea of the effectiveness of non-active care early on, as well as the idea that pregnancy is a time of change and transition which can make us feel uncertain about many aspects of our lives. It is this uncertainty, the sometimes excruciating experience of not 'knowing', which leads to acceptance of, and over-emphasis on, the 'risk' element of pregnancy and birth. This leads us to demand more 'stuff' in the name of good care. Much of the accepted routine in maternity care is built around 'curing' women of their uncertainty, instead of supporting them through it. There is a way forward, a way out of the cycle of fear, helplessness and blame and alternative healthcare can be a significant stepping-stone along the path.

CHAPTER 2

A STATE OF HEALTH

The vast majority of pregnancies are normal and healthy. The vast majority of women begin their pregnancies believing that they are healthy and that pregnancy is a normal life event. But somewhere along the way the perception of what is healthy and what is normal changes.

If most pregnancies are normal, why do so many women experience them as abnormal? In part it may be because of the deep emotional challenges which pregnancy brings. There are also unfamiliar physical signs of pregnancy. Often women are simply expected to cope with these without any information about why they occur and without any advice on how to lessen their impact. While the physical complaints of pregnancy are not a sign that you are ill, they can make you feel as if you are. This can be very distressing for the woman who is used to taking her health more or less for granted.

The next, and perhaps most important, reason why pregnancy may feel so abnormal is that it is often managed in hospitals and clinics – places where sick people go. The atmosphere in which most antenatal testing is done, with its emphasis on illness and abnormality, can provoke enormous anxiety and loss of confidence among women.

Such an atmosphere also provokes fear among doctors and midwives. They may, without being aware of it, pressure women into accepting all the routine tests rather than deciding upon each according to its relative merits. Women who exercise the right to choose, or refuse, are often viewed as 'difficult'. They disrupt the schedule and don't fit into the well-planned, though not well-proven, style of maternity management.

In spite of all this, and even if it takes you into some new and unfamiliar territory physically, psychologically and emotionally, there are some good reasons for never losing sight of the fact that pregnancy is a state of health.

REDEFINING HEALTH

Whatever your time of life, the idea of optimum health must always encompass more than the mere absence of illness or uncomfortable physical symptoms. It must also include a sense of emotional, social and spiritual well-being. Good health, in short, is a state of wholeness.

If this seems like a tall order at any time of life, but particularly during pregnancy, perhaps it's because in modern healthcare we focus on the body to the exclusion of all else. The reason for this is because we know, within certain limits, how to study the body and how to ascertain what effect illness, drugs and surgery have on our physical health. It is much harder to study the effect of these things on the mind and emotions – and even harder to study the interplay between mind and body and the impact this has on patterns of health and disease. Not surprisingly, our focus in pregnancy is equally narrow, concentrating on its physical side to the exclusion of its other more subtle components. But even as we accept that these things matter, we are still missing a crucial point about our definition of wholeness and health.

Hawaiian mothers believe that if they vomit a lot during pregnancy it is a sign that their child will grow up to be a good provider. If the mother can afford to waste food in this way, they reason, it must be because the child will always provide more.

As a general rule, good health, like so much in Western society, is defined by what is appropriate and normal for a fit, young male. But females, because of their ability to conceive and bear children, have a rather more complex biology than men. Medicine has long wrestled with the 'problem' of female biology and the way that, for instance, women tend to react differently to certain drugs and surgical procedures. Medical researchers are often ethically obliged to exclude women of childbearing age from their studies. Because of this there is still, surprisingly, much we do not know about the true pattern of female health and disease. What is clear though, is that a woman's health needs, particularly while pregnant, must be measured by a different standard.

In the same way that women can bleed without being injured, they can during pregnancy, experience a bafflingly wide range of symptoms without actually being sick. At this time some of the major body systems – digestive, hormonal and nervous – come under greater stress. The 'symptoms' of pregnancy such as nausea, constipation and exhaustion are expressions of the body's attempts to adapt and rebalance itself. They aren't always comfortable, but neither are they signs of illness.

A great deal of medical research has gone into the issue of what makes a pregnancy normal or abnormal. Norms have been established, but not to reassure women of their normality. Instead, they are used as measures in the search for the abnormal.

At the same time, many practitioners are relying on outdated or incomplete information to guide them in their work. New information about what is normal, and how miraculously well a healthy woman's body functions during pregnancy, has been slow to be incorporated into medical textbooks. Furthermore, the norms expressed in the tables and graphs of obstetric manuals don't usually take into account differences between ethnic groups, nor can they include individual family history. A small woman carrying a small baby will still be told as a matter of routine, 'your baby is not growing well', because norms also don't take into account the body frame of the respective parents.

Obstetrically defined norms don't allow for healthy variations on normal either. Although various methods of testing have provided us with increased knowledge about fetal development and the biochemical changes which women experience, there is a price to pay, often in the form of extreme anxiety when individual babies and bodies don't follow the accepted 'norm'.

For instance, it is fairly common for an early ultrasound to pick up an anomaly – something not usual, but also not likely to be threatening. A good example would be a 'cyst' which the sonographer identifies on the baby's kidney or elsewhere. In this case 'cyst' is a descriptive word. It may not be a cyst at all. It's just something which isn't usually there, and which will in most cases disappear as the baby develops. However, once this anomaly has been picked up, it must be followed up. More scans will be scheduled. Both mother and baby are now 'patients'; and even if her baby is born healthy and well, the mother may live with nagging doubts about the health of her child.

Another example would be the measuring of women's iron levels. Far too many women today are being diagnosed as anaemic or borderline anaemic. This diagnosis ignores the fact that pregnant women's bodies use nutrients more efficiently and will be absorbing more iron from their food than they would in their non-pregnant state. It also ignores several other biochemical facts: a woman's blood volume does double during pregnancy but the 'ingredients' of the blood, the red and white cells and the plasma,

Portuguese and other sea-faring cultures have a belief that a baby born with a caul, that is, still inside the amniotic sac, is good luck. Some believe that such a child has magical powers and others see it as a good omen meaning the child will not die by drowning.

do not increase proportionately. The largest increase is in plasma – the fluid which transports red and white blood cells around the body.

A pregnant woman may actually have more iron circulating in her body, but testing methods used primarily on non-pregnant individuals do not allow for the uneven increases in blood constituents.

BODY CHANGES, BODY CHALLENGES

Once pregnancy is confirmed, a woman enters arguably one of the most startling and exciting periods of her life, and one in which she may become more body-aware than ever before. Many are surprised to find that almost no part of their body remains unchanged by pregnancy. Some of these changes, such as dry eyes, tingling fingers and legs and sinusitis, are temporary. Others, like stretch marks, will be with her for life.

The sort of 'normal' changes associated with pregnancy will vary from woman to woman. Reactions to body changes can also vary. What causes concern in one woman may be nothing more than a mild inconvenience to another. What they all have in common is their normality and frequency.

The fact that such changes are 'normal', however, is of little consolation if you are feeling ill and uncomfortable. Happily, there is much you can do on your own to help relieve uncomfortable symptoms. More detailed suggestions for dealing with many common complaints are made in the section of this book dealing with therapies. Where possible, the general advice here should be used in conjunction with any alternative method you choose. Also, remember that many of the symptoms you experience will be less intense if you are able to make the time to rest during each day. This is especially true during the first few months of pregnancy, when nausea and fatigue are common occurrences.

Backache

As pregnancy progresses, the additional weight you are carrying can put your lower back under stress. Over the months your pelvic joints will be loosening up in order to facilitate labour and the structure which normally supports your back becomes less stable and less supportive. In addition to spinal pain, some women also experience sharp pains which begin in their sacroiliac joints (the joints which lie on either side of your tailbone) and shoot right down the leg, making walking and moving difficult.

Stay off your feet when you can. Sacroiliac pain can feel worse when you lie on your back, so try resting in a different position, well-supported by pillows if necessary. Back pain can also be the result of postural problems. Some find the progressive shift in their centre of gravity hard to adapt to and end up arching their backs and thrusting their bellies out to compensate. Pay regular attention to how you are standing and sitting and try to keep your pelvis tucked under you.

A good exercise for this is the pelvic tilt. To do this, lie on the floor, breathe in and as you exhale press the small of your back against the floor. Once you've mastered this movement, practising the same thing standing up will help improve your posture. In addition, when you can, avoid high-heeled shoes, which will only make maintaining a stable posture more difficult.

Bleeding

Slight bleeding or spotting during pregnancy does not necessarily indicate a miscarriage. Around 10 per cent of women will experience

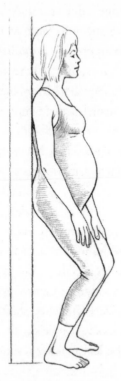
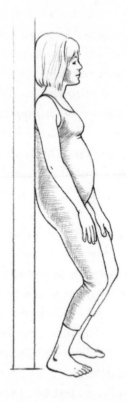

▲ Pelvic tilt – standing

Stand with your feet a little way from the wall and comfortably apart. Bend your knees a bit so that your bottom, back and head are all touching the wall.

Push your lower back firmly against the wall, tightening your stomach muscles and tilting your pelvis forward and slightly up. Your bottom will leave the wall but your shoulders should still be against it. Hold this position for a count of four, then relax. Repeat several times.

For each position make the tilting movement gentle. Exhale as you tighten the muscles.

▼ Pelvic tilt – lying down

Exhale as you press the small of your back against the floor. Hold this position for a count of four, then inhale and relax your spine. Repeat several times.

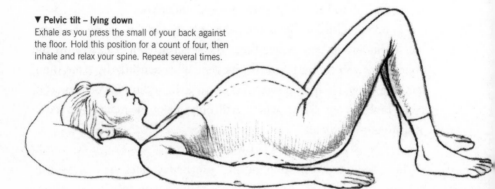

some bleeding during the first 28 weeks of pregnancy, and slightly fewer after that time. When it does occur it can often be linked to the time when you would normally be having a period. Bleeding may also occur around 14 weeks, when the placenta takes over hormone production from the corpus luteum (the part of the ovary which produces several different hormones including progesterone, which stimulates the lining of the uterus to grow).

Less common is the bleeding from an ectopic pregnancy. In an ectopic pregnancy, the embryo gets 'lost' and implants itself elsewhere than the uterus, usually in one of the fallopian tubes. This potentially more dangerous bleed usually occurs around 6 to 12 weeks and is accompanied by one-sided abdominal pain. Bleeding is caused by a rupture of the tubes and must be addressed with surgery to terminate the pregnancy and repair the tube.

After 28 weeks, bleeding and pain can be caused by the placenta prematurely peeling away from the uterine wall. This rare condition is known as placental abruption and is accompanied by continuous pain. You will be losing blood internally so if you suspect this, get to the hospital immediately since your baby's and your own life will be at risk.

Finally, bleeding very near to term can occur if you have *placenta praevia* – where the placenta is covering the cervix. As the cervix dilates (and this process can begin before labour) the placenta can be torn. Because of this, women with placenta praevia are often advised to have a caesarean before term although this is not always necessary (*see* chapter 6 for more information).

There is not much you can do about any of these types of bleeding. Doctors often advise that early bleeds require complete rest. Rest and contemplation are an important way to deal with the profound emotions caused by an early bleed. However, there is little good evidence that resting will avert a possible miscarriage. If you are more comfortable being up and going about your business you should be able to make this choice without being made to feel guilty. Keep the homeopathic remedy Arnica 30C in your medicine chest and take this hourly for up to four hours until the bleeding stops or you can be seen by your practitioner.

Candida

Fungal infections (also known as thrush or yeast infections) can be aggravated by the hormonal changes of pregnancy, which alter the acid/alkali balance of your vagina.

It is normal to experience increased vaginal secretions during pregnancy, but if your vulva becomes red and irritated and you have a white, cottage cheese-like discharge it is a sign of vaginal candida. It is best to clear this condition during pregnancy since your baby can become infected at birth.

Antifungal pessaries and creams will be ineffective after a while, so instead of treating the symptom, treat the cause. Possible triggers include overuse of antibiotics, stress and previous use of the birth control pill, but the strongest link is with diet. If you are prone to candida infections it is particularly important that you remove all acidic and sugary foods and refined carbohydrates from your diet. In some women dairy products are also a trigger. Instead, make sure your diet is based on whole foods and includes plenty of immune-boosting garlic, onions, turnips, cabbage and plain, live yoghurt.

Candida loves warm, moist atmospheres, so wear loose cotton underwear which allows air to circulate. If you regularly use bubble baths, stop. They will irritate the area further (and are implicated in recurrent urinary tract infections in mothers and babies). Also, no douching (*never* in pregnancy) or vaginal deodorants, and switch to white, unscented toilet paper.

Early signs of vaginal candida can be treated with plain, live yoghurt. Before going to bed, insert a few teaspoons into the vagina. Repeat this each evening until the symptoms improve. Caught early enough, the friendly bacteria in the yoghurt will multiply and devour the candida. Calendula cream or tincture will help ease external irritation. In addition, you might persuade your partner to be tested for candida since you can become reinfected through sexual contact.

Constipation

Hormonal changes during pregnancy will make food move more slowly through your digestive system. Although generally hormonal in origin, constipation can be made a great deal worse by a poor diet. Stress can also make it worse and if your symptoms are really severe, it may be worth considering whether you have a food allergy or intolerance. Constipation can also be caused by iron supplements.

Instead of laxatives, increase your intake of fibre. Not the kind you find in wheat bran, but the more bowel-friendly kind you find in raw vegetables, fruits, oat bran and rice. This fibre is water-soluble and will aid the passage of foods through the gut. Wheat bran is an irritant and, because it is not water-soluble, it can make your stools dry and harder to pass. For breakfast, try including fruits such as figs and prunes – but not the processed kind which can be high in sugar.

Massage is not only pleasant and beneficial for the mother – it may also have effects both direct and indirect on the baby. Jamaican midwives believe that they can 'shape the baby' by giving regular abdominal massages with castor oil. The Japanese also practise hara massage, a special massage for the belly believed to stimulate the fetus and encourage it into a favourable head-down position.

Drink plenty of fluids. The more you drink the more efficient your system will become at flushing out toxins and other impurities. Try drinking a cup of hot water flavoured with a squeeze of lemon juice just before, or with, your meal. If this does not appeal, try a herbal tea such as camomile, fennel or ginger. Eating small, unhurried meals throughout the day will help your system process food more efficiently.

Massaging your belly in a clockwise direction is also helpful. Gentle massage (with or without aromatherapy oils) can be carried out by yourself or your partner and can be very pleasant as well as effective.

Cramps

You can get muscle cramps almost anywhere in your body during pregnancy but the most common site is the calves. Often these painful spasms seem to come out of nowhere, and although individual spasms may only last a short time, they can be very severe. For quick relief stretch the muscle by extending your heel and bringing your toes towards you.

Cramp can be the result of the extra weight you are carrying. Stretching in bed in the morning and pointing your toes can also bring on quite severe muscle spasms. Cramps may also be caused by salt or calcium deficiency and circulation changes, so the best prevention is to make sure that you take regular exercise and watch your nutrient intake. Your diet should include plenty of calcium and magnesium-rich foods (*see* appendix 2, page 290) and you should salt to taste.

Cystitis

This urinary infection can strike quite suddenly and is caused by an inflammation of the bladder. You will know when you have it because urinating can become excruciating, producing a burning pain, and you will have the urge to pee even if there is nothing in your bladder.

Cystitis can occur alongside other vaginal infections such as candida. Since both are linked strongly with diet you should investigate food allergies as a possible cause.

You can prevent attacks by wearing cotton underwear and not getting too chilly. Avoid spicy and sugary foods and alcohol. Drinking *unsweetened* cranberry juice is very helpful. If you cannot find this, try some of the other cranberry-based remedies available in healthfood shops. Your best option during an attack, however, is to drink plenty of water. Putting a teaspoon of bicarbonate of soda in your glass of water will help relieve symptoms.

If you take early action, you will probably be able to avoid antibiotics. However, if you do need to resort to antibiotics, make sure you take supplemental probiotics, such as acidophilous and bifidobacteria, at the same time and eat lots of plain, live yoghurt.

Fatigue

No matter how energetic you are, at some point pregnancy will take its toll on your energy levels. There is no complicated remedy for exhaustion. When you are tired you must rest. In the end, the best way to prevent exhaustion is to listen to your body and learn your new limits.

As pregnancy progresses you may find it more difficult to sleep.

Finding a comfortable position may be difficult and you may need to get up frequently to urinate. Aches and pains may bother you more and interrupted sleep can result in extreme fatigue. Tiredness can also be linked to your emotional state, for instance if you feel anxious or depressed.

Developing new ways of approaching rest and relaxation will help. Taking catnaps during the day will make a big difference to your energy levels – it will also get you into a good habit for after birth, when you will need to rest when the baby rests.

Being physically run down can produce fatigue, so in addition to regular periods of rest, make sure you are eating well. Avoid junk food, especially those high in sugar and caffeine. Regular exercise can actually help relieve tiredness and aerobic exercise is a particularly good choice.

Fluid Retention

Water retention in pregnancy is common and, on its own, rarely a sign that anything is wrong. Only when it is combined with high blood pressure and protein in the urine is it a possible sign of pre-eclampsia. Water retention is especially noticeable late in pregnancy, when you may find that your rings and bracelets no longer fit properly.

Hot weather, prolonged standing, and fatigue can make puffiness in the fingers, ankles, calves, feet and face more pronounced.

One side-effect of water retention is Carpal Tunnel Syndrome. This is when increased supply of fluids to the extremities causes swelling and pressure on the nerves and blood vessels which pass through the wrist canal (known as the carpal tunnel). When this happens you may experience numbness, tingling and even pain in the hand, fingers and sometimes the arm. The condition usually improves after birth.

Your body needs the extra water volume to cope with all the extra substances which are floating around in it (such as waste products created by your baby) so don't take diuretics. Your kidneys are under enough strain already and these will only cause problems. A good wholefood diet and regular exercise will promote the elimination of excess water and help reduce puffiness. You will also need to make sure you get plenty of rest each day. Try supplementing your diet with natural diuretics such as garlic, raw onions, apples, red grapes or grape juice.

Carpal Tunnel Syndrome can be worse in the morning due to fluids accumulating in your hands overnight. Try holding your arms over your head for a short while to drain off excess fluids. Gentle massage to the wrists and hands will also help ease the pain.

EMOTIONAL CHANGES ARE NORMAL TOO

Worries about yourself, your relationship and your baby are to be expected as you prepare for parenthood. Ambivalence, feelings of anxiety and depression are natural to pregnancy, as natural as they are to any other major life transition. One minute you may feel confident and joyful, the next down in the depths of tearful despair for reasons you can't even articulate.

Perhaps in another age some of these feelings would have been met with faith in a higher authority such as God or Nature, or sound advice and support from a mother or friend. Today a woman's feelings of confusion and despair are dismissed, rather cruelly, as nothing more than 'hormones'. More commonly, because we find it so hard to accept that negative and positive feelings can co-exist in pregnancy, labour and beyond – and that women do not need to be 'saved' from this paradox – we use what we believe to be the certainty of screening to address women's uncertainty. Many doctors truly believe that simply reassuring a woman her baby is all right is the happy solution to unhappy feelings during pregnancy. This, of course, ignores the fact that the mother may not be all right and may be very unhappy for reasons which do not directly relate to her baby.

Certainly a woman might fear miscarriage. She may fear for the baby's well-being and be grappling silently with the dilemma of termination versus the realities of raising a handicapped child. But equally, once a baby is on the way, other issues come sharply into focus. If she and her partner were just getting by financially before, the reality of a baby will highlight the need for more money and more 'things'. Her home may seem suddenly smaller. She may feel less efficient at work, or suddenly realize that she actually doesn't like her job very much, but with a baby on the way feels trapped into staying there. The dynamics of her intimate relationship will change, even before the baby arrives. A woman and her partner may be seeing new sides to each other for the first time. If she lives far away from family she may be worried about lack of practical support once the baby arrives.

Anxiety may also be tied up with a shift in self-perception. Women today, as always, function in multiple social roles. Taking on yet another role, that of mother, will involve a period of anxiety. Because so many women are led to believe that it's unreasonable to be unhappy if you have a healthy baby, anxieties and fears are often expressed instead as over-concern for the baby's well-being.

Constant feelings of anxiety and depression should be taken seriously, since they are a sign of unmet needs. These needs could be for emotional support and reassurance. Some may stem from your childhood or more recent past (never underestimate the way pregnancy and impending motherhood can trigger long-suppressed fears and memories). Equally, they could be more practical, such as the need for more and better information. Many a rational woman has been driven to the edge of despair trying to find out simple information about her options for maternity care!

When you are depressed or anxious it is likely that you feel less inclined to take care of yourself. If you can, make greater efforts to do so; ensure you take time out to rest and to eat since exhaustion and low blood sugar will adversely affect your mood. Instead of bingeing on chocolate, however, make sure you eat nutrient-dense whole grains, fruits and vegetables which will maintain your blood sugar level. Taking regular exercise will release helpful endorphins into your system. These natural mood-lifters, combined with the rhythmic movements of many exercises, can reduce feelings of depression and worry. Also, consider seeing a birth counsellor or psychotherapist. Talking things over, even if only for a few short sessions, can help put things into perspective.

But most of all, remember that as long as you are well-supported and doing the best you can for yourself and your baby, it's OK for emotions to be mixed. If one day you hate being pregnant, resent being slow or heavy or vague, your baby will not suffer emotional damage as a result. The key is to acknowledge your feelings without making value judgements about them or yourself. Because things change so rapidly during pregnancy, tomorrow you may feel entirely different. You may feel beautiful, glowing, sexy and on top of things again. Try to enjoy the ride.

Headache

Pregnancy does not raise your risk of developing headaches. However, since a number of women feel under a greater amount of stress at this time, stress-related headaches are not uncommon. Headaches are also more likely on hot days when the extra weight and the extra blood you are carrying will make it harder for you to keep cool. Ironically, some women who suffer from regular migraines find that their headaches disappear during pregnancy!

The best way to deal with headaches is to do all you can to prevent them occurring. Try to anticipate stress at home and in the workplace and, where possible, do what you can to limit your exposure to stressful situations. Learn to listen to your body and when it says you have had enough – stop. Pregnancy can exaggerate adverse reactions to some foods: if you are able to link your headaches to a type of food it is best to remove it from your diet.

Heartburn

Another effect of increased circulating hormones in your body is the softening of the valve between the oesophagus and stomach. When this happens, foods and gastric acids can be regurgitated. These can irritate the lining of the oesophagus, causing a feeling of pain and a sharp, burning sensation in the chest. As your uterus grows it can aggravate things further by putting pressure on your stomach. Heartburn can follow a rushed meal; it can also follow an emotional upset. Food allergies are also a potential cause.

Eating small, frequent meals is a good idea. The wisdom of this will become more apparent as you get bigger and your stomach gets squeezed into a smaller space. Don't eat too late at night – give yourself at least two hours to digest your evening meal. Digestion begins in the mouth, so relieve the burden on your stomach by chewing your food well.

The kinds of food you eat may also be important. Cut out spicy, greasy, sugary or acidic foods. Some women find that not drinking with a meal helps, since sometimes this can dilute digestive juices. Instead, try sipping a herbal tea such as fennel after a meal to aid digestion but stay away from coffee and tea, since they can increase stomach acidity.

Insomnia

Your sleep patterns will change during pregnancy and the occasional sleepless night is not uncommon, especially late in pregnancy. If insomnia becomes a regular feature of your pregnancy, however, your health will begin to suffer.

Often the cause is emotional. During a busy workday you may not have time to think about impending parenthood and how it will affect your life. At night, when things are quiet, you may find that worries crowd your mind. You may feel depressed and anxious and all these feelings can interfere with your ability to drop off to sleep.

Try to avoid sleeping pills, which do not benefit you or your baby. Talking to someone – either your partner, a self-help group, your midwife or a counsellor – is the best way to deal with the worries that keep you awake.

If you feel physically uncomfortable and this is keeping you awake, try being creative with the pillows on the bed. If necessary, invest in a few more so you can prop various parts of your body up at night. As pregnancy progresses you may feel hotter, so make sure the room is well-ventilated.

Although you should not eat a main meal too close to bedtime, a light snack just before retiring can help you avoid night-time hypoglycaemia. The brain needs a constant supply of glucose even at rest and a drop in blood sugar signals the body to produce chemicals that stimulate sugar release. The resulting rise in blood sugar can actually wake you up. Finally, regular exercise – but not just before retiring – can improve the quality and duration of sleep.

Nose-bleeds

Spontaneous nose-bleeds are the result of the greater amount of blood circulating in your body. They may come on when you feel particularly

TURNING 'SICKNESS' INTO HEALTH

The nausea women feel, particularly in early pregnancy, is usually called morning sickness. It's not a very apt name since it doesn't always happen in the morning and it isn't really a sickness. Feelings of nausea, occasional vomiting, tiredness and lethargy are as common as they are uncomfortable. For most women these symptoms disappear after the first few months. However, for some, especially those expecting twins, they may last throughout pregnancy.

There are many contributing factors to nausea during pregnancy. Some are physical: low blood sugar, low blood pressure, hormonal changes, nutritional deficiency (especially in vitamin B6 and iron), or nutritional excess (especially spicy, sugary and refined foods). If nausea reappears during the last few weeks of pregnancy it can be because the growing uterus is putting pressure on the stomach. But there is also an emotional side to nausea. Women who are carrying unwanted babies, or who feel in some way resentful about the pregnancy, seem to experience nausea more severely than those who do not.

Nausea accompanied by relentless vomiting requires medical help since this can dehydrate and rob the woman of essential nutrients. Otherwise, try these self-help measures:

• Take two or three teaspoons of apple cider vinegar (not any other kind) in warm water first thing in the morning.

• Make a warming tea by pouring boiling water over a teaspoon of freshly grated ginger root. Sweeten with honey if your prefer. If you are out of the house and can't brew up, any food item containing ginger should help. Some women swear by stale ginger ale, others prefer the crystallized ginger available in some specialist cook shops. Still others use it liberally in cooking in both sweet and savoury dishes.

• Acupressure can be very effective. Studies show that pressure on the pericardium 6, or P6, point can provide relatively quick relief from nausea, though it may not help to reduce vomiting. To find this point place your hand palm up and measure two thumb widths above the most prominent wrist crease; P6 is just above this point,

in line with the middle finger). Some chemists sell wrist bands which stimulate the P6 point and claim to help relieve nausea. These have been shown to work for some women.
• Numerous studies have shown that deficiency in vitamin B6 is at the root of many cases of nausea. Try taking at least 25 to 50mg daily as part of a B-complex supplement.

stressed, since your blood pressure will also rise during these times. The condition usually improves after birth.

In the meantime they can be stopped by using a cold compress on the bridge of your nose while keeping your head back. Some women find that a small amount of petroleum jelly rubbed inside the nostrils helps stop the bleeding. Try to avoid blowing your nose too hard, as this can also bring on a bleed.

Restless Legs

This is an uncomfortable condition which produces a strange, crawling sensation in the legs, rather like having an electric current running through them. It occurs mostly in the early evening and at night when you are resting, making your legs feel uncontrollably jittery, giving you an irresistible urge to move around. Restless Leg Syndrome can make relaxation and even sleep difficult, since it produces repeated and uncontrollable leg shakes. The condition usually disappears after birth.

There are several contributory factors to this condition. Hypoglycaemia is one and overuse of caffeine is another. The combination of the two has been shown to make symptoms worse. Anaemia is a factor, so make sure you eat plenty of iron-rich foods. Adequate levels of folic acid and vitamin E may also be helpful. Some people find that regular exercise helps alleviate the condition. Warm baths before retiring are also helpful.

Sinus Congestion

Sinusitis in pregnancy can often be caused by a swelling of the mucous membrane inside the nostrils and sinuses. For some women, especially in later pregnancy, the condition can become chronic.

Sinus problems usually improve after birth but in the meantime you may have to learn to breathe through your mouth. If this makes your mouth feel dry, especially at night, keep a glass or bottle of water handy and take frequent sips. Try also keeping your lips moisturized with lip balm or cream. Sometimes nasal congestion is associated with food allergies and a good nutritionist will be able to guide you in this matter. In the meantime you might also want to consider cutting down on foods which can increase nasal secretions, such as dairy products. Although these are often considered essential in pregnancy, other good sources of protein and calcium will ensure that you are adequately nourished while relieving pressure on your sinuses (*see* appendix 2, page 290).

Stretch Marks

Some women get stretch marks and some don't. Although it is more common in women of Celtic extraction, there appears to be little rhyme or reason for their appearance. They are not necessarily linked with weight gain, there is very little convincing evidence that there is much you can do to prevent them appearing, and once they have appeared you can't simply rub them away with creams.

Whenever your body gets bigger more rapidly than your skin can adapt to, stretch marks will appear. Pregnant women are not the only ones who get them; they are quite common, for instance, in both male and female body builders. Although they fade over time and are non-threatening to a woman's health, many women feel deeply emotional about their stretch marks. The more you feel that pregnancy shouldn't change your life, the more stretch marks seem to mock you and remind you that your body and your life have changed permanently. Accept them, and take what few steps you can to limit their appearance.

Steady weight gain throughout pregnancy will take the strain off your skin. Make sure your diet is rich in vitamins C and E, both essential for maintaining skin tone. Some women swear by cocoa butter and there are

Pain – The Dress Rehearsal

Are the discomforts of pregnancy random, meaningless biological happenings? The answer is probably not. How you cope with the various symptoms you experience says a lot about how you will cope with labour. In spite of what you may have heard, coping has little to do with bravery or 'pain thresholds', and a lot to do with personal resources.

Before a woman even has the chance to come to terms with being pregnant she will be asked 'Are you going to have pain relief?' (That's usually the second question; the first is 'Have you had your scan yet?') The focus on pain is both terrifying and frustrating and leaves many women feeling as if they simply don't have the resources to cope. But one reason why labour pains are so scary is that we do not see them in the context of the whole pregnancy. As a result, more and more women feel afraid of this unfamiliar, unstoppable pain, which they see heading straight for them like a derailed locomotive.

A more positive approach would be to look at labour pains as one end of a spectrum of body pains and discomforts with which you have already coped well. You could even say that digestive problems, leg cramps, Carpal Tunnel Syndrome, bloatedness and exhaustion are a 'dress rehearsal' for the bigger, less predictable, pain of giving birth. They are the regular little pains which prepare your body for the main event.

Although it may seem difficult, now is the time to reframe your thinking about pain. How you perceive these day-to-day aches and pains and how you deal with them provides a framework for dealing with the pain of labour, so now is a good time to look at how you manage pain yourself. Do you pamper yourself? Are you the type who grins and bears it? Do you run to the medicine chest for a quick fix? Look also at how your partner copes when you are not feeling well. Is he supportive? Does he think you are just complaining? Does he ignore you? Does he feel unable to help?

If you can both learn to deal with the discomfort you are feeling now in an appropriate, sensitive and non-aggressive way, the approaching pain of labour will not seem so daunting.

Nothing can really prepare you for the pain, or rather the sheer physical force, of labour. But managing the discomforts of pregnancy through natural, alternative methods will help to improve your confidence. Try to congratulate yourself each day on how well you have coped so far, and use this to strengthen your ability to cope later down the line.

a number of good formulations on the market. It is unclear whether a special stretch-mark formula is genuinely better than a simple, solid cocoa-butter preparation. Lotions will feel lighter on the skin but solid cocoa butter has the advantage of providing a wax-like barrier which locks moisture into the skin. Vitamin E oil rubbed daily into the abdomen, breasts and thighs may also be of benefit.

Varicose Veins and Haemorrhoids

Increased blood volume during pregnancy puts your veins under pressure. In addition, hormonal changes relax the muscular walls of the blood vessels. This action makes it more difficult for your veins to move blood from the lower body back to the heart. The increasing weight of your uterus will put more stress on the pelvic veins, and if you are experiencing constipation this can also interfere with your pelvic circulation. As a result, blood may pool in the lower body and you may get bulging, painful varicose veins on the legs, vulva or rectum.

Varicosities tend to run in families. Pregnant women who have to stand for long periods of time (for instance at work), who sit for long periods during the day and those expecting twins may also get them. Varicosities of the vulva will usually disappear after birth. Those in the anus or legs may or may not improve, depending on what action you take to prevent or relieve them during pregnancy.

Avoid constipation and exercise regularly to improve your circulation. Rest with your legs up as often as you can and when seated avoid crossing your legs. Wear support stockings and avoid squatting or standing for long periods of time.

To reduce swelling, try a cold compress or ice pack on the affected area(s). Likewise, a cool sitz bath (a shallow bath which just reaches your legs and/or bottom) may help improve circulation.

The way your child is born will also affect whether or not piles improve – a good reason to avoid strenuous 'pushing' (the baby *will* come out without it), forceps and ventouse deliveries.

ADDRESSING CONCERNS ABOUT YOUR BABY'S HEALTH

It's fair to say that most women perceive antenatal screening as a good thing. They perceive it as an important part of their care and don't always think of less invasive procedures such as blood tests or ultrasound as 'tests' at all. Instead, they see them as a way of addressing any concerns they might have about their baby's health. There is absolutely nothing wrong with antenatal testing as long as it is used appropriately and consciously by women and their practitioners. Unfortunately, most testing is done with both practitioner and mother on auto-pilot.

In unravelling the question of appropriate testing, a good place to start is with a question: why do so many healthy women feel at risk?

There is no simple, single answer. On a cultural level, routine testing, whether it's the seemingly trivial ritual of weighing a woman or the more invasive amniocentesis, reinforces some powerful insecurities. Since women are rarely brought up to believe in the perfection of their bodies, pregnancy can be a time of great uncertainty. After all, how can the female body, so widely perceived as imperfect, dysfunctional and largely out of control, create a perfect baby?

From a clinical point of view, some of the 'risk' factors, as defined by medical norms, exist mainly to increase women's 'risk' of anxiety. A woman will be told she is 'at risk' of a damaged baby or a difficult birth if she is, among other things: under 18 or over 36; having her first child or has had four or more children; uncertain of the date of her last menstrual period; has had a previous small baby or a previous large baby; has had a previous caesarean; has had a previous long labour or a previous short labour; has had a previous forceps delivery; was overweight or underweight before conception; too short (under 5 ft); has put on too much or too little weight during pregnancy. The results are ludicrously narrow parameters for defining a woman as 'low risk'. Not surprisingly, many normal, healthy women carrying normal, healthy babies end up being labelled as 'high risk', even though only around 10 per cent of those allocated to high risk groups actually experience the predicted problem.

Another reason for high anxiety is the conditions under which many women are expected to make decisions about their care. Usually options are presented early on, in the unfamiliar and disquieting setting of a hospital or clinic. The woman may be suffering from morning sickness, or extreme tiredness. She may be under pressure from family or friends, who may themselves have experienced pregnancy and birth as a negative event or who are fearful of the process. They may be pushing her to take action, take tests, in fact do anything, to ease their own anxiety about the coming birth.

The combination of an unfamiliar environment, unfamiliar physical symptoms and pressure from her nearest and dearest may make a woman feel as if there must be something wrong with her or her baby. She may agree to tests which in another state, physically and mentally, she would not otherwise consider necessary.

Is This Test Really Necessary?

Don't just agree to routine tests. *Decide* about them. As the chart on pages 36–7 shows, each one has merits and risks which should be weighed up carefully.

In a perfect world, a woman's decision to choose or refuse a test, and everything which follows it, should be based on good information. Yet, most women's knowledge about antenatal screening is still very limited. Sometimes this is because practitioners convey little information or present it in a way which is misleading. Many doctors have such great faith in antenatal testing that they believe that discussion of the pros and cons is a waste of their already limited time. Some believe that 'too much' information will only worry or confuse mothers. This assumption is not borne out by fact; recent studies have shown that offering women more information does not confuse them or increase anxiety.

When considering special tests such as ultrasound, CVS or amniocentesis, remember that a diagnosis is not the same as a cure. Once diagnosed there is often little that can be done to correct a problem save offering the mother a termination. If you are one of the 30 per cent or so of women who would not consider a termination on any grounds, then there is little point in you going through the battery of tests on offer antenatally.

Before you panic, or let anyone around you panic, consider what the real risk is. There are a few simple questions you should ask of your practitioner, and yourself, before agreeing to any antenatal test. They are:

• Does this test *directly* benefit my baby? If so, how?
• What are the documented risks of the test? To myself? To my baby?
• How conclusive is the result?
• Can the condition you are testing for be cured or corrected either now or when the baby is born?
• How does knowing about this condition early benefit my baby or me?
• Would the outcome be the same if I didn't have the test?

Making Sense of Tests

Test	When offered	Useful for	Possible risks
Urine A non-invasive test using a specially coated dip-stick	First and subsequent antenatal visits	Can confirm pregnancy. A sample may also be analysed for evidence of infection and traces of protein which may indicate pre-eclampsia.	None, but dip-stick tests are notoriously difficult to read accurately. Two different practitioners may see two different results. Ask for a second opinion if the test indicates something wrong.
Blood Requires the drawing of a small amount of blood	First antenatal visit	Confirming blood type and rhesus status. Increasingly woman are also asked if they wish to be tested for HIV status.	Most blood tests are straightforward. However, a number of factors, including flu virus, rheumatoid arthritis and having more than one child can produce false positive HIV results. Those who test HIV-positive should take independent advice and ask for a second opinion.
Blood pressure Non-invasive measurement of the flow of your blood as it enters and leaves your veins	First and subsequent antenatal visits	Checks primarily for abnormally high blood pressure. The number on top – the diastolic pressure – is when the blood enters the vein. The number on the bottom – the systolic pressure – is when it leaves. The combination of the two measurements provides a snapshot of your circulatory health, *at that moment in time*.	None, but blood pressure can vary from day-to-day and from hour-to-hour. Normal blood pressure during pregnancy is between 100/60 to 125/80. In labour it can go up to 140/90 without indicating a problem. Many things can influence the results such as how tired or stressed you are. When blood pressure rises only in the clinic, this is called 'white-coat hypertension'. If you suffer from this, you can ask to have your BP taken at home where you feel more relaxed.
AFP/double/ triple/triple-plus test Blood test which requires the drawing of a small amount of blood	Between 16 and 18 weeks	Tests for a limited range of disorders, primarily Down's syndrome and spina bifida. Standard AFP test looks for a single 'marker', or chemical, in the blood; the double test, two 'markers' and so on.	Terribly inaccurate. Only detects 50 per cent of affected babies and only 10 per cent of those estimated to have an affected baby actually do. Results can be made more inaccurate if your pregnancy is further advanced than the doctor believes, if you smoke, if you had an early bleed, if you are black and if you are carrying a boy or twins. In retrospect, many women regret having this test since they then become pressured into having a second, more invasive test to confirm or deny the results of the first.
Ultrasound High frequency sound waves are bounced off your baby. The echo returned to the main machine is interpreted as a picture	Standard scan is performed at about 16–20 weeks. Some women are offered more throughout pregnancy	Looks for a range of abnormalities including Down's, spina bifida, neural tube defects, heart conditions and other abnormalities of the internal organs. At best, only picks up 80 per cent of a limited range of abnormalities.	Ultrasound is an unproven technology which has been associated with the rise in learning difficulties among children. There is mounting evidence that it alters brain function and may also damage soft tissues. It is linked with an increased risk of miscarriage in women prone to miscarriage. Repeated ultrasound scans are no better than a single scan in improving outcomes, so consider limiting your and your baby's exposure.

Test	Description	When	Risks and notes
Fetal heart monitor A form of ultrasound which is used to listen to the fetal heart	Contrary to popular belief, this is not a microphone. It is a complex ultrasonic device which scans the baby in the womb and interprets what it finds in the form of a heartbeat.	Used every antenatal visit unless the mother requests a less invasive monitoring such as a Pinard or stethoscope	Risks are hard to assess and are perhaps best examined as part of the mother's total ultrasound exposure. If you are uneasy about exposing your baby to ultrasound you should ask to hear your baby's heartbeat with a stethoscope or have it monitored by a hand-held Pinard.
Nuchal scan Early ultrasound scan	Looks for a special fold of skin behind the neck. Thicker folds are thought to be an indication of Down's syndrome.	Usually performed before 12 weeks	No evaluation has been made of how safe early scans are for the baby. Recent studies have concluded that the Nuchal scan is no better at detecting abnormalities than the standard scan and may carry more risks for the baby.
Transvaginal scan Ultrasound through the vagina	A probe which bounces ultrasonic beams off the baby is inserted in the vagina. Because it is closer to the baby doctors say they get a clearer picture.	Can be given at any time	The amount of ultrasound your baby will receive will be many times greater since it will not have the advantage of being protected by your abdominal muscles and fat. This is an intimately invasive test which carries all the same risks of other forms of ultrasound, perhaps more, as well as the risk of infection from having a foreign object inserted into the vagina. Should not be used on women with placenta praevia or a cervical stitch.
Chorionic Villus Sampling (CVS) Laboratory analysis of tissue removed from the developing placenta	A needle is inserted into the womb through either the cervix or the abdomen. The aim is to remove a small part of the chorion – the cells which will eventually develop into the placenta. These cells are analysed for signs of abnormalities such as spina bifida and Down's. Results will also reveal the baby's sex.	Performed at between 9 and 13 weeks	You will be removing a tiny part of the placenta – a risk which some mothers feel is too great. Babies who have had CVS have more breathing difficulties, raising the issue of whether the test may create health problems rather than solve them. The risk of club-foot also rises with CVS. This is a special test to be reserved for those at high risk of having a child with an abnormality.
Amniocentesis Laboratory analysis of fluid removed from the womb	A needle is inserted in the womb via the abdomen. It is used to withdraw amniotic fluid which will then be analysed over a period of several weeks. Used to detect Down's, spina bifida and neural tube defects. Results will also reveal the sex of the child.	Should be performed at between 16 and 20 weeks	Must be used with ultrasound otherwise the risk of the needle puncturing the baby is many times increased. Women may experience spotting and cramping afterwards and older women have a greater risk of miscarriage from the procedure. May cause breathing difficulties in the baby. Not always conclusive; some lab cultures fail and then the test must be done again. Many women find amnio uncomfortable and scary. Best reserved for special situations.
Pelvic X-ray X-ray of the pelvic bone structure	Used to assess the internal dimensions of a woman's pelvis to see whether there is enough room for the baby to come out. Occasionally used to confirm congenitally misshapen pelvis.	Usually offered towards the end of pregnancy	Very inaccurate and now abandoned by many hospitals as a means of assessing the dimensions of a woman's pelvis. Chances are your baby is not too big to come out. The risk of exposing your baby to X-rays is well documented and includes an increased risk of childhood cancer.

CHAPTER 3

GUIDELINES FOR A HEALTHY PREGNANCY

On its own, your body is supremely capable of creating the perfect environment for a healthy baby to grow in. But this doesn't mean that you have no conscious contribution. Many aspects of our modern lifestyle conspire to make your body's job more difficult. These include stress, financial pressures, poor dietary habits, sedentary lifestyles and a polluted environment. To help your pregnant body do its task well, your job is to protect it from the onslaughts of modern life. Because mother and baby are a single unit, whatever you do to maintain your body's health will also benefit your baby. Good health practices can ease even the most uncomfortable symptoms of pregnancy as well as ensuring better long-term health for your child.

One of the most important aspects of self-care is adequate nutrition. For as long as we have been studying human health it has been obvious that, to a large extent, we are what we eat. A great deal of research has accumulated to show that what a mother eats while pregnant can have a truly dramatic effect, not only on how her baby grows while inside her but also on the long-term health of that child.

A plethora of studies shows that hypertension, coronary heart disease, thyroid dysfunction, diabetes and the propensity toward other autoimmune diseases and degenerative diseases such as Alzheimer's – the possibilities of which cannot be detected by any antenatal test – are all programmed into a baby while still in the womb. What determines the programming is maternal nutrition during that time.

We also know that the miscarriage rate goes up in women who are not adequately nourished. It is ironic that we now have many drugs and methods for helping women who find it difficult to conceive, but we still ignore the most obvious solution: change your diet, put on some weight and try again.

Once pregnant, many women assume that as long as they are getting a fairly good diet everything will be fine, but this may not be the case. If the mother is on a moderately good diet the baby may be fine, but she could begin to feel increasingly tired, unwell and unable to cope. If the mother is on a poor diet, her health and that of her baby may rapidly begin to deteriorate.

A very poor or restrictive diet can quickly begin to have detrimental effects on the baby, chief among which is poor fetal growth. Evidence shows that during famine conditions the average birth weight can go down by as much as 550g (1lb 3oz). It would be easy to argue that the term 'famine conditions' applies only to poor countries and not the affluent West. Nevertheless, around a third of the babies born in the UK are born into families who are defined as 'poor'. Also, dietary restriction, whether self-imposed out of a fear of getting 'fat' or medically directed, can have exactly the same effect, subjecting healthy women to famine-like conditions which can adversely affect their babies' growth.

Some women reading this might wonder whether having a small baby is such a bad thing – surely it will make the birth easier? But the overwhelming evidence tells us that low birth weight babies are the ones who find labour the most distressing, who have the lowest health scores after birth, who are at greater risk of dying in the first six weeks of life and whose long-term physical and emotional health prospects are among the poorest. If a mother has fears about growing a big baby or having a difficult birth these must be addressed with rational information and the reassurance that a) women seldom make babies that are 'too big' to come out, and b) the size of your baby has little to do with the kind of labour you will experience.

Although it is usual to scan babies regularly for birth defects, doctors often omit to tell mothers that under famine conditions the rate of birth defects also goes up. Observation of traditional cultures shows that it only takes one generation of eating a typical Western diet – high in fats, sugars and salt and low in fresh produce and complex carbohydrates – to begin to adversely affect their children's health.

WHAT SHOULD YOU EAT?

Diet is arguably the most important aspect of maternal self-care and yet this is one thing which women rarely receive any coherent advice about. In fact, when women think of diet and pregnancy they usually think in terms of restriction. They think of what they can't eat – soft cheeses, shell fish, wine and beer – and what the doctor or midwife has told them they should cut back on – salt, coffee, tea, spices and even water. They think of food cravings and aversions. Or they focus on nutritional magic bullets such as iron, folic acid and magnesium, instead of total nutrition.

YOUR BABY'S GOOD TASTE

Not only does your food provide the building blocks for your baby's growth, it also provides, quite literally, a taste of the environment it will be born into. Several studies have shown that amniotic fluid becomes flavoured according to what the mother eats. In this way it is thought that babies become acclimatized to the food preferences of their culture.

We know that babies have a natural sweet tooth. In one study of babies who were growing poorly, the mothers' amniotic fluid was sweetened with a sugar solution in an attempt to get the babies to drink more of it – and they did! Less appealingly, it has recently been discovered that babies can, in the same way, taste the tobacco that their mothers breathe in when they smoke cigarettes. Scientists now believe that the taste and the craving for tobacco is passed on from mother to infant in this way.

Rarely do they think of what they can and should include in their diets or that food during pregnancy can become meaningful and enjoyable. It may never occur to them that a pregnant woman's heightened sense of taste and smell can make meals more interesting. Or that while they are making life more interesting for themselves, they are also making it better for their baby.

But as important as nutrition is, we are also more than the sum total of what we eat. Outside influences such as the amount of stress we are under and the amount of pollution we are exposed to will also influence how well we assimilate and utilize nutrients. However, when you are pregnant your body will generally be using food more efficiently, so if your appetite is larger than before, make sure you are eating with a purpose. Junk food binges are as unwise as alcohol binges.

Common sense dictates that you should avoid refined and processed foods, in particular those which have a high sugar content, since sugar has an immediate depressive effect on the immune system, leaving you vulnerable to illness. Fatty foods and those which list additives, preservatives, flavourings, aromas and stabilizers among their ingredients should all occupy only a small part of your diet, if they are part of it at all. It may also be wise to limit your consumption of red meat (if not in frequency, in portion size), replacing it in your diet with oily and/or deep-sea fish and poultry. Stimulants such as coffee, tea, cocoa and cola, all of which contain caffeine, should also be used in moderation, if at all.

Pregnant women are often advised to increase their daily intake by 300 to 500 calories. But women don't eat calories, they eat food. Hunger, not calorie counting, is likely to be your best guide to appropriate eating during pregnancy. Nevertheless, certain guidelines do apply.

In practical terms you should aim to have the following foods daily:

- 5 portions of whole-grain products – cereals, breads, rice, etc.
- 2 servings of green vegetables
- 2 eggs
- 2 servings of dairy – preferably organic
- 3 pats of butter or three tablespoons of unrefined vegetable oil (olive, sunflower, grapeseed)
- 1 citrus fruit or similarly high vitamin C food such as berries, tomatoes, cauliflower, potato and sweet potato
- 2 extra servings of high-protein foods, particularly fish and poultry, but also cheese, nuts and pulses
- Plenty of non-caffeine drinks such as water, herb teas and grain coffees made from barley or chicory. Fruit juices are fine too, but limit or dilute these because they can be high in sugar

In addition, five times a week you should include:

• a yellow or orange coloured fruit or vegetable, for example cantaloupe, sweet potato, papaya, carrot, mango, orange, apricot or squash
• an iron-rich food; traditionally offal such as liver and kidney. However, because of the toxins which commercially reared animals ingest, you should only have offal from organically raised animals. Otherwise consider suitable alternatives such as beans, nuts, asparagus, small portions of red meat, molasses, oatmeal and dried peaches, apricots and prunes.

Remember that a diet for pregnancy is not a diet for life and that the recommendations above are simply guidelines. They can, and should, be adjusted to suit your individual tastes and preferences. In fact, more than any prescribed eating plan, variety is the key to getting all the nutrients you need.

While you are pregnant go ahead and eat for two but remember that eating for two doesn't refer to the quantity you are eating – but rather its *quality*. If you restrict anything at all, make sure it is fast-foods with empty calories.

One final recommendation is that the closer a food is to its natural state the more nutrients you will get out of it. Thus fresh is optimum, frozen is acceptable, canned is useless. Eating produce in its raw state is ideal, particularly in the warmer months. However, if you like your vegetables hot, remember to steam or cook them only very lightly to preserve their nutrients. Lightly cooked vegetables and fruits are particularly suitable during the winter.

We think of the humble banana simply as a good source of potassium and quick energy, but other cultures see it as a 'cooling' food which can lower both the physical and emotional temperature of the mother. In Thailand, pregnant women eat bananas to ensure their babies are born with a 'cool' temperament.
In Chinese culture, mangoes and pineapples are considered too 'hot' and are thought to encourage miscarriage.

If you are prepared to eat seasonally, very fresh, organically grown produce is now more widely available. Apart from having no harmful pesticides, this food will have been picked fresh and arrive with relative speed at your table. This is in complete contrast to the produce in the supermarket which can be stored for months before being put on display, depleting it of essential nutrients.

GM Foods

Increasingly, news headlines about genetic modification leave many of us anxious and confused about the food we eat. We now have the technology to alter the most basic building blocks of life. Unfortunately we have not conducted the studies necessary to prove or disprove the safety of GM foods, in either the long or the short term. We are unaware of whether GM foods can, for instance, cause damage to a vulnerable fetus at certain stages of development. GM foods don't taste better and they are not cheaper to buy; they have, however, been implicated in increased resistance to antibiotics and the growth of super bugs. They have also been linked to an increased incidence of allergies.

Food can either be genetically modified itself, or contain genetically modified ingredients or derivatives. The issues are very complex but if you are concerned you might consider avoiding or limiting:

Tomatoes (and tomato purée) were the first GM foods to be sold. In the US you can buy fresh tomatoes which have been genetically modified; in the UK you can only buy purée made from these tomatoes. Watch out for ready made foods such as pizza which may use GM tomato purée.

Soya has been modified to resist weed-killer. In the US, supplier of most of the world's soya, GM soya and unmodified soya are not kept separately and processed foods may contain both. Soya is present in most baked and pre-packaged foods in several forms: oil (often just labelled vegetable oil), vegetable fat, flour, lecithin, vegetable protein.

Maize has been modified so that it contains a bacteria toxic to a common crop pest. Maize is used as a grain, as corn (or maize) flour, corn meal, corn starch, corn syrup, dextrose, glucose, fructose, xanthan gum, maltodextrin, and as corn oil. Be aware of products such as chocolate bars and sweet drinks which contain sugars derived from maize.

Cheese can be made with a GM enzyme called chymosin instead of traditional rennet. Chymosin is used in many vegetarian cheeses and increasingly in hard cheeses for general consumption.

Enzymes are used in a large number of products including drink, bakery goods and dairy products. Manufacturers are not obliged to include these on the product information.

Canola, or rapeseed, is mainly used as an oil. Some crops now contain human genes.

Yeast which has been genetically modified has been approved for making bread, but it is difficult to know the extent to which it is used in bakery products.

Vitamin B2, known as riboflavin, is now widely produced from genetically modified micro-organisms. It is generally added to breakfast cereals, soft drinks, baby foods and diet foods.

E numbers indicate preservatives, flavourings and colourings. Watch out for E101, E101a, E150, E153, E161c, E322, E471, E621, all of which may be GM derivatives.

To spot GM foods you will have to become a reader of labels. Even this will not guarantee that your diet will be GM-free. Labelling laws in the UK and in the US are very confused and seem to exist mostly to protect the manufacturer rather than the consumer. There is no requirement to label a product which may contain GM ingredients, flavouring or additives, and only a very few volunteer this information. In the UK, several supermarkets have announced that they have removed, or are in the process of removing, GM foods (but not always derivatives, so check carefully) from their own-brand products. Nevertheless, the best way to avoid GM foods is to eat as much organic and freshly prepared (by you, in your home) food as possible.

Avoiding Environmental Hazards

The environment you live in will also have an impact on your and your baby's health. Our world is becoming increasingly polluted. We ingest pesticides, fungicides and antibiotics with our food, we breathe in lead and other harmful chemicals every time we leave the house. Many of the things we associate with making our world and ourselves more 'civilized', air fresheners, fertilizers, household disinfectants, hair dyes, even fluoride toothpaste, contribute to a growing toxic load on our bodies. Increasingly research is showing that environmental toxins may be responsible for a growing number of health problems among children.

Nobody can avoid all pollution, but it makes sense to try to reduce the total toxic load on your body whenever possible. Simply being aware of some of the sources of indoor and outdoor pollution can provide you with the wherewithal to make subtle changes in the way you live and work, should you wish to.

Toxic Metals

Among the most potentially harmful substances to a developing baby are toxic metals such as lead, cadmium, aluminium and mercury – environmental pollutants which can enter the body through being inhaled or through the food we eat. The greater the mother's exposure, the greater the risk to her child. The reason is that while these pollutants build up slowly in your body over time, they are slow to clear from your system. Some, like mercury, never leave the body.

Lead is found in most water supplies as well as in the emissions from car engines and factories. It can get into your system through breathing in polluted air, it can also be absorbed through the skin. Women should be aware that if their partners work in jobs where they are exposed to high levels of lead (plumbers, painters and motor mechanics, for example) the women can become contaminated with lead through their partners' semen. Once you are pregnant you might consider using a condom to avoid lead being absorbed into your body from your partner's seminal fluid.

Lead can also be in the food you eat since plants and animals may also have been exposed to these pollutants during their growth. Lead contamination has been associated with deformed and dead sperm, infertility, repeated miscarriage and stillbirth. It may also be linked to low birth weight. High levels of lead in pregnant women can predispose their children to dental caries.

To reduce your intake of lead, consider having a reverse osmosis water filter installed. If this proves too expensive, make sure you run the tap a minute or two before you use the water from it for cooking or drinking.

A healthy diet will help combat the effects of lead. Make sure your diet is rich in foods with vitamins A, C (including bioflavonoids), D and E, and minerals iron, calcium magnesium, manganese, selenium, chromium and zinc, as well as protein and fibre. Eating lots of fresh garlic can also help combat the effects of excessive lead.

Cadmium has been linked with both stillbirth and low birth weight. The most common source is cigarette smoke – yours and others. It is also present in drinking water, certain plastics and paints (especially those with a red or orange colour), enamelled cookware and some insecticides. In addition, there can be cadmium in refined cereal products such as white flour and bread, alcohol, oysters, gelatine, some canned foods, pigs' kidneys from animals treated with a worm-killer containing cadmium, and caffeinated drinks such as cola, tea and coffee.

To avoid cadmium overload, avoid cigarette smoke, even the passive kind. You might consider changing your enamelled pans as well, since cadmium can be released during cooking. Keep your diet low in refined foods and be aware that alcoholic drinks may contain cadmium as a preservative – another good reason to cut down or quit during pregnancy.

Aluminium is toxic in high quantities. It may even cause the deterioration of placental function. Every time you cook in an aluminium saucepan you expose yourself to this toxic metal. If the food you are cooking is acidic (such as apples, spinach or rhubarb) it can release more metal into the food. Many pressure-cookers are made with aluminium and this cooking method can also concentrate the metal in your food. Keep foods heated in tin foil or served up in freezer-to-oven foil trays to a minimum.

Aluminium is also used as an anti-caking or bleaching agent in foods you use every day such as salt, milk substitute and flour. It may also be present in high levels in your drinking water. Antiperspirants contain aluminium and although the manufacturers claim that this is unlikely to be absorbed into your blood stream, this has not been proven. It is also present in antacids.

To minimize your exposure to aluminium, steer clear of cooking utensils made from this metal. Make sure foil coverings are not touching fatty foods during cooking. Avoid bleached white flour products and foods containing the additive 556 (aluminium calcium silicate), E173 (aluminium–CI77000) and 554 (aluminium sodium silicate). Food rich in manganese will help counteract the harmful effects of aluminium.

Mercury also interferes with placental function. It affects the central nervous system and children with high levels of mercury may also be prone to health disorders such as allergies. There is mercury in our drinking water and you may also ingest it by eating tinned fish such as tuna. Weed-killers and fungicides also contain mercury. But perhaps the biggest source of mercury is the fillings in your teeth. It is now widely accepted that dental amalgam leaks over time, leaching toxic metal into your body.

One answer is to have your metal fillings replaced by composite ones. This can prove to be expensive – although there is no rule which says you have to do it all at one time! It is best to have fillings removed before conception. Don't attempt to have them removed during pregnancy, since airborne particles of the drilled mercury can be inhaled and get back into your system via your lungs. Instead, do what you can to reduce your mercury intake, for instance by avoiding canned foods, especially fish. There is some evidence that eating plenty of garlic will help limit mercury absorption.

Balancing Exercise and Rest

Pregnancy places a great many demands on your body. When you are pregnant, your body will change in ways you may not even be aware of. For instance, your heart will eventually double in size and the amount of blood in your body will also double. When one study compared the heart health of pregnant women to non-pregnant women it found that the cardiovascular fitness of the pregnant women was greater than that of the non-pregnant women, even though they took significantly less exercise. Just being pregnant, it seems, is enough to give you an all-over body workout.

Nevertheless, for healthy, well-nourished women (and subject to only a few restrictions) exercise, particularly in early pregnancy, has real benefits. A regular exercise programme will help relieve some of the transient discomforts of pregnancy such as constipation, haemorrhoids and insomnia. It will improve muscle tone and endurance, both of which are needed during labour. Exercise improves circulation, and those who engage in regular exercise tend to have more stable blood pressure. In the later part of pregnancy regular, gentle exercise may be of benefit to women who are told they have gestational diabetes, since it will help the body use insulin more efficiently. The deep, regular breathing which is part of many exercises will enrich your blood with oxygen and will be as good a practice for labour as any prescribed breathing practice.

BETTER FOR THE BABY TOO?

Almost anything which promotes good health in the mother will benefit the baby. Better circulation, in particular, will mean that the placenta is enriched with nourishing blood and the baby may well enjoy and benefit from the rhythmic rocking motion of some exercises. If the mother is combining exercise with meditation such as in yoga, the hormones released in her relaxed state will also 'relax' the baby.

But as with everything else in pregnancy there can be a downside to engaging in very vigorous exercise, particularly in late pregnancy.

Lengthy aerobic exercise at this stage may reassure the mother about her health and her body, but sometimes it does not benefit the baby. Muscles need blood to work and during vigorous exercise blood is diverted away from non-active muscles to those which are working the hardest. Late in pregnancy, exercising too hard can draw essential blood away from the uterine muscle and this can have an impact on the baby's health, compromising fetal growth and increasing the risk of pre-term labour. Given this, late pregnancy may be a time to consider other, less demanding forms of exercise.

For busy women, exercise is often incorporated into daily activities, for instance, taking the stairs in early pregnancy instead of the lift, or walking to the shops or the post office instead of taking the car. This is as legitimate as any other form of exercise. However, some women genuinely enjoy the social aspect of prenatal fitness programmes – getting together with other women at various stages of pregnancy and being part of a group. What is more, there are psychological benefits in taking part in exercise which is strictly a leisure pursuit and which doesn't involve mundane household chores and running errands for other people.

Which Exercise?

Your best choices include walking, swimming, tennis, cross-country skiing, dancing, weight training, sailing, yoga and Alexander Technique. These last two choices are particularly appropriate since they will improve your flexibility (both physical and emotional) and during labour flexibility will be more helpful than strength.

A helpful hint for choosing an exercise is to think about how your body feels and choose according to your needs. For instance, if you feel that your increasing weight is making you less flexible and light on your feet, swimming and especially yoga can do you a world of good. If you feel lethargic in early pregnancy, getting your heart rate up with an aerobic exercise can help move things along.

Be aware, though, that some exercises can make things worse. For instance, plunging yourself into a cold swimming pool may wake you up, but if you are prone to leg cramps, it could bring them on.

In addition, consider the following guidelines:

• Generally speaking, pregnancy is not a good time to take up a new, vigorous sport; staying with the familiar may be more advisable.

• Your heart rate should remain at comfortable levels and be monitored to avoid getting overheated, dizzy or short of breath. For women who engage in aerobic exercise, avoiding expansive arm movements should ensure that your heart rate does not rise too rapidly.

• You may want to pay more attention than usual to body temperature. Your baby cannot control its own body temperature and relies on you to be its thermostat. Not overheating or becoming too cold are sensible precautions. Try to stay hydrated during exercise and sports activities to help keep your body temperature within normal range.

• Jarring movements may be more risky during pregnancy and you should take special care to protect your lower back, which will come under increasing stress as your pregnancy progresses. Likewise, running and anything which places a high impact on the muscles and skeleton, as well as activities which involve being off-balance or suddenly changing direction, should be avoided late in pregnancy.

• Avoid scuba diving; the oxygen is too rich for your baby's system and the increased pressure on the systems of both mother and baby may starve the baby of necessary oxygen.

The danse du ventre *(womb dance), otherwise known as belly dancing, with its pelvic rocking and rippling of the abdominal birthing muscles, is believed to have been practised not only as a rite through which the Mother Goddess was worshipped but also as a form of gymnastic preparation for childbirth.*

• In early pregnancy bicycle riding may be beneficial but on today's roads it can be hazardous – a helmet won't protect the most precious and vulnerable part of your body. Also, as you get heavier, your centre of gravity will shift and you may not feel as stable on a bicycle as you once did.

• If you are participating in organized events make sure your teacher is experienced in working with pregnant women, whose needs are different. Specially dedicated classes are often best.

Finally, when the uterus experiences excessive stress it will start to contract. Some forms of exercise, particularly those in which the woman is using her legs, may cause uterine contractions due to stress on the womb. These mostly harmless contractions can be hard to notice unless you are very tuned into your body.

However, a contraction, even a mild one, can be a sign that the exercise is too intense and needs to be halted. Like any other muscle, when the uterus contracts it feels hard. By placing your fingers just below your diaphragm, it is possible to palpate the uterus to contraction. An experienced midwife or doctor can help you learn what this type of mild contraction feels like so that you can recognize it in the course of your exercise regime.

Exercising the Pelvic Floor

Your pelvic-floor muscles may not show, but the more toned they are the more efficient they will be at aiding your baby's passage into the world. Doing your pelvic-floor exercises also means that you are less likely to suffer any prolonged physical problems in this part of your body after birth.

The pelvic floor isn't really a floor at all but a complex structure of muscles which supports everything in the pelvic cavity, including the uterus, bladder and rectum. The easiest way to identify your pelvic-floor muscles, if you have not already done so, is to interrupt a stream of urine. These muscles also contract spontaneously during sexual intercourse, intensifying pleasure for you and your partner. Awareness and control of your pelvic-floor muscles is also helpful during labour, since you will need to release them as your baby passes through the birth canal.

The muscles around the opening of your vagina and your anus can be contracted together or separately. To contract the muscles around the vagina, imagine that you need to urinate but must hold it in. The 'holding' involves a contraction of the pelvic-floor muscles. Contracting the muscles around the anus involves the same kind of 'holding' action.

You should aim to do your pelvic-floor exercises twice daily, in sets of 20 to 30. You can do them in bed first thing in the morning and last thing at night or, if you're really motivated, in the car or on the bus or anywhere you feel inclined. At first, some women find this exercise difficult. They don't see the point or find that their muscles tire easily and they can't keep them contracted for very long. Some find that when they try to tighten these muscles, they end up holding their breath and tightening other muscles in their shoulders, neck and arms instead. But as with all exercise, it gets easier to do with practice and you will find that you will be able to relax and eventually hold the contracted muscles for up to a count of ten.

Taking Time to Rest

Every period of exercise should be balanced by a period of rest. This does not necessarily mean sitting around doing nothing. Rest time can be used to meditate and actively reflect. Any hobby which completely absorbs you will also be restful, since it will take your mind off things and allow you to focus completely on a single task.

Not unnaturally, some pregnant women find that the quiet times are the most difficult. Instead of relaxing their minds and communing with the baby, they find they are overcome with nagging fears and doubts. You may find yourself worrying about whether you can cope during labour, whether you will be a good mother, how much time you can afford to take off around the time of birth, whether you will be able to meet the demands of your new baby, and what your partner's reaction to new parenthood will be.

All of these worries are normal and legitimate, but don't be deluded into thinking that if you just make a greater effort you will find some sort of rational answer to it all. Pregnancy is a process. It is a journey into the unknown. Apprehension about the unknown is natural and learning to deal with the unfamiliar is good practice for all the future unknowns which crop up once you become a parent.

If anxiety and worries come up when it's quiet or during meditation don't be too hard on yourself. Acknowledge them briefly and then try to let them go. Switching off for half an hour will make no difference to solving the riddle of impending motherhood and you will emerge more refreshed for having done so. If your worries persist, it is generally a sign that you don't have enough information about whatever you are worrying about. Perhaps you haven't allowed yourself to fully explore what's worrying you. Or it could be a signal to talk to someone and ask more questions.

If you are worried about your baby or have questions about your pregnancy and find that your midwife or doctor is too busy or does not give you satisfactory answers, go elsewhere. Several useful groups exist to help provide information and support to pregnant women. Groups such as AIMS and the NCT provide telephone support as well as producing a wide range of booklets and leaflets.

If your anxieties centre on you and your partner, now is the time to open the channels of communication. The insights gained in moments of calm and reflection can be a useful starting point. Share your feelings in the best way you can and encourage your partner to do the same. If you can take a weight off your shoulders in this way, it can sometimes feel as good as if you've had a long, long rest.

In an active world, it's easy to forget that there are other forms of 'cardiovascular activity' which are important. Making room in your heart for this new little person is a big job, one which can only be done in moments of reflection and calm.

CHAPTER 4

MOTHERHOOD AS A SPIRITUAL JOURNEY

There are touch-points in every life which entreat us to change and grow; to mature and act like adults, to take responsibility for ourselves, our lives and the people we love. Pregnancy is a touch-point.

The Ancient Chinese believed that pregnancy was a spiritual practice which lasted for nine months. During this time the mother was expected to spend her time in quiet contemplation and prayer. She would surround herself with pleasant things mental, emotional and spiritual. This gave the mother inner strength and solid ground to stand on. And since the mother's physical and spiritual well-being has a direct influence on the fetus, it also provided the baby with a strong foundation.

Looked at from the perspective of Western culture this view of pregnancy may seem quaint. Yet we know that a baby in the womb responds to its mother's emotions. For instance, studies have shown that babies move less and even grow less well when their mothers are anxious. Some psychotherapists believe that the experience – good and bad – of being inside our mothers remains with us for life and that it is possible to remember those experiences through the act of rebirthing.

Not every pregnant women welcomes such information. Perhaps this is because nearly every pregnant woman has had a moment when she wished she was not pregnant, or that life could go back to the way it was before the coloured dot on the home pregnancy test changed her life so completely.

Some, however, don't feel threatened by the idea that the baby can 'read' their thoughts. Instead, they believe, as some therapists do, that the baby can benefit from experiencing its mother's full range of emotions and that such an experience forms the basis of the child's emotional education.

Of course, it's not just the child whose life is profoundly affected by the time spent inside its mother. For many women, carrying a child, being aware of the pulse of a new life pulsating within them, is the catalyst for re-evaluating their place in the world. It becomes a time to review priorities and decide the extent to which they will allow the conventions and values of the world at large to influence their personal behaviour.

Your Philosophy of Life

Apart from acquiring practical skills, some prospective parents become acutely aware of the need for a kind of spiritual re-education, which includes a review of their priorities and their philosophy of life.

If we accept that the experience of pregnancy is an extension of our experience of life then certain questions about life as we experience it become relevant to experiencing pregnancy in an authentic way. For instance: *'What's important to me in this life?'*, *'What are my principles?'*, *'What do I care about?'*, *'What am I willing to stand up for?'*. These are the questions which form the basis of your individual life philosophy. Such questions also provide the basis for all the choices women make about themselves, their babies and their care during pregnancy.

Perhaps you've never taken this sort of personal inventory before. It may seem daunting even to contemplate it. But if you are up to it, the most useful way to begin is to get a sheet of paper (or two) and just write out your 'philosophy' about life. Typically, this would include some statement as to why you think we're here on Earth, what it is that you believe we are supposed to do while we are here, what you think is important in life (and what is not important), and which values of your society you agree with and which you do not.

For those who wish to take the exercise further, below are some other elements which go into making an individual life philosophy. You can use any of these (though you don't have to use all of them) or you may simply choose to write out what you feel inside yourself. Either way, don't expect the answers to come easily or necessarily even to make sense immediately. Some answers may seem simple and straightforward to you, others may not. You may want to contemplate the issues raised over a longer period of time. Having begun to think of these things, don't be surprised if any problems which you are experiencing begin to take on a new dimension – either more complex or suddenly simpler than you thought.

Beauty What is beautiful to you? How important is it in your life?

Behaviour How do you think we should behave in this world?

Beliefs What are your strongest beliefs?

Choice What do you think about its nature and importance?

Community In what ways do we belong to each other and what do you think our responsibility is to each other?

Compassion Why do you think it's important and what are the best/most appropriate ways to express it in daily life?

Confusion or ambivalence Is it a normal part of life? How much do you think we need to learn to live with?

Death What do you think about it and what do you think happens after it?

Events What do you think makes things happen and how do we explain this to ourselves?

Evil Is there such a thing? How do you identify/define it?

Free will Are things preordained or do we have free will?

God/Supreme being Do you have a concept of One? If so, what do you think the Supreme Being is like? What does the Supreme Being mean in and demand of your life?

Heroes/Heroines Who are yours? Why?

Human What do you think makes somebody truly human?

Individuality In what ways do we stand alone? What does it mean to be an individual?

Love What do you think is its nature and importance? What qualities do you relate to love (for example, grace, forgiveness, trust, etc.)?

Morality What is it? Which issues concern you most?

Principles Which ones are you willing to stand up for and which do you base your life on?

Purpose Why do you think we are here on this earth? What would you say is the purpose of your life?

Reality What can you say about the nature of reality?

Sacrifice What in life is worth sacrificing for and what would you be willing to sacrifice?

Self What do you believe about yourself, your ego, selfishness and selflessness?

Stewardship What do you think we should do with God's gifts to us?

Truth What is the truth and in what areas is it most important to you?

Values Which are the ones you hold most dear, sacred and important?

Violence What is violence? Is it a physical, mental and/or emotional phenomenon? Is it ever justified?

Looking over such a list, you may still be wondering, *what's all this got to do with being pregnant?* Yet, when you are carrying another life inside you issues such as stewardship, love, faith, ambivalence, sacrifice, death, individuality and free will are with you every day. They are with you when you decide about antenatal tests, when you think ahead to labour, when you experience ups and downs with your partner and in the middle of the night when you wonder 'Who am I?' and 'What resources do I have to cope with parenthood?'

One of the reasons why the subjects on this list seem so overwhelming is because we rarely take the time to think about what they mean to us and to look for the places in which they influence our lives. If you've never done such an exercise before it can be quite an eye-opener. Often people find, for example, that although they thought they had strong principles they can suddenly think of rather too many times when they have compromised these. Or it dawns on them that they have never really given death and dying much consideration, or that their views about death have changed dramatically since becoming pregnant.

Your individual life philosophy isn't just for your benefit. The fact is that conception, not birth, is the beginning of parenthood. While it is common to feel that as parents we have only a limited influence over our children's lives, in fact our influence is enormous. As a parent you will be passing on your philosophy of life both consciously and unconsciously. It will form the basis of your child's moral education. Spending

According to Mexican Indians it is the mother's anxiety – often felt as knots in her stomach – which can make knots in the umbilical cord.

some time now thinking about who you are and what is important to you will improve your chances of handing on the values and beliefs that you intended to share with your child.

FACING THE PAST

We give birth as we live. Our beliefs about ourselves, the way we've experienced the world, manifests in our lives and in the way we order our birth experience. The experience of midwives and doulas (birth sisters) around the world is that when a woman enters birth (whether it be for the first time or the fourth) with a lot of unexamined emotional baggage, when she is fearful for reasons she can't articulate, birth tends to be many times more difficult. When a woman is assisted to understand her own beliefs and to express what is important to her, she is able to change her birth outcome. There are many kinds of emotional baggage, but two which are very relevant to birth are a history of sexual abuse and a previous unhappy birth experience.

Life with abusive parents can take its toll on you even as an adult. Women who have been sexually abused may be particularly vulnerable when they become pregnant. They may have deep-seated anxieties about their bodies and themselves as sexual human beings. The body changes, the aches and pains of pregnancy and birth can bring back unpleasant, frightening memories of abuse which will need to be worked through with the help of a counsellor, if at all possible. If they are not, birth can end up being a catalogue of further abuses. Even simple antenatal examinations may bring up terrors and labour will seem simply insurmountable.

When we speak about the sexuality of birth we must look at it as part of the total picture of a woman's sexuality and not as an isolated example. If the highest estimates are true and one in three women in the UK has been the victim of sexual abuse, then is it any wonder that birth, as a sexual experience, is so frightening? A woman who cannot release herself into the sexuality of sex because of the devastating emotions and memories it brings with it, will certainly be unable to release herself into the sexuality of birth.

Sometimes it is the recent past which needs clearing. Memories of a traumatic birth experience can overshadow the next pregnancy, making it difficult for the woman to go forward and reinforcing her fears about herself and her body.

Should any kind of birth result in a live baby, women are told they should be grateful. Yet a difficult birth, whether the baby lives or dies, can take a long time for a mother to fully recover from. Long after any physical scars have healed, emotional scars may still be weeping and sore to the touch. Some women carry bitterness and resentment over their birth experiences with them to the grave.

Although a previous difficult birth may seem, on the surface of things, greatly different from a legacy of childhood abuse, at heart the two are the same. Often a gross abuse of trust has taken place which can adversely affect your life and relationships from that point on. The process for overcoming abuse, no matter where or when it took place, is much the same.

When working through the experience of a previous traumatic or difficult birth or if you are overcoming a legacy of childhood abuse, consider:

• The past does not have to repeat itself. You can't change what happened to you in the past, but you can alter the course of your future.

• Talk about it to friends and family, but perhaps most importantly to a sympathetic and skilled therapist or counsellor. If you are angry, then be angry. If you are sad, cry until you are all cried out. It is important to surround yourself with people who understand that your feelings are facts and will not simply brush you aside with glib assurances that you'll be fine and that all that matters is a healthy, live baby.

• Do you need to speak to your abuser? Do you need to speak to the doctor or midwife who oversaw your previous birth? If you have issues with someone, now may be a good time to have your say.

• Would it help to write your experience out as a story? This could be your story and the story of your child. What comes out in moments of creative expression can also be very healing.

Remember it is often important to clear the past before you can step into the present or even contemplate the future. Having done so, many women find a renewed interest in themselves, in their lives and in the experience of being pregnant and giving birth.

WORKING WITH DREAMS

When you are pregnant you may experience very vivid dreams. Indeed, some pregnant women are deeply disturbed by their dreams, especially when they feature giving birth to a handicapped child or losing the baby in a crowd and not being able to find it again. Some women experience violent dreams which reflect the violent emotional changes they try to suppress during the day, and fear that this means that they will be violent or 'bad' parents. Still others experience idyllic, reassuring dreams which help to counterbalance the fears which they may have during waking hours.

Dreams are a dialogue which you have with yourself. The biggest mistake people make is to assume that the images featured in their dreams have literal meanings. Thus, what appear to be disturbing images are often interpreted as warnings about the future. But dreams do not speak to us directly; instead they employ the language of metaphor. If you are really interested in finding out what your dreams mean, first put away any books you have on dream symbolism. Try not to associate specific images with specific meanings: snakes are not always phallic and finding money on the ground doesn't mean you are going to come into good fortune. Instead, focus on what the image or images mean to you personally and try to bear in mind that often in dreams each of the characters represents a facet of your own personality.

While a dream about your best friend or partner may actually have something to do with them and your relationship with them, it is also likely to say a lot about the part of your personality which is most like them. A good example would be a dream about your best friend who is single and childless. She sits in a comfortable chair, leaving you to stand exhausted under the weight of your pregnant bulk. Perhaps in reality your friend is having trouble adjusting to your needs now that you are pregnant, but equally there may be a part of you which does not recognize and respond to your changing needs adequately.

Your dreams during pregnancy are the most direct way to tap into your own feelings and into the development of your baby. They are to be welcomed as a way of working through the changes you are going through. One good way to keep track of them is through a dream diary. Any old notebook will do. If you can, make time to write down your dreams each morning and then write down any feelings or impressions you had upon waking.

A number of themes crop up again and again in the dreams of pregnant women. While it is impossible to give blanket interpretations of all of these, here are some of the most common:

Dreams during pregnancy have significance to many cultures. Some are thought to be predictive: among the Maoris of New Zealand, there is a belief that if the mother dreams of a human skull she will give birth to a girl, but if she dreams of feathers her child is a boy.
Among the Bataks of Sumatra, if the mother suffers from bad dreams it is taken as a sign that she is being haunted by bad spirits and needs extra protection from her husband during the night in order to prevent the baby from becoming upset.

Giving birth to an animal

The kind of animals you give birth to in your dreams may change according to how advanced your pregnancy is. If you look at pictures of embryos up to about 12 weeks they do look rather like lizards. While your baby is inside you it is in what you might call an animal or instinctive state – concerned mostly with life's basic needs, such as food and comfort. As your baby's body develops, and its senses become more refined, it is quite natural for the baby animals in your dreams to change from reptiles to cuddlier, more 'human' animals, such as puppies and kittens. Although it may seem a strange dream, it could be viewed as a kind of update on your baby's progress. This interpretation can be modified, however, according to your perception of the animal in question. If you are very afraid of dogs or snakes then it is the fear and how it relates to your baby which will need to be explored.

Losing the baby in a crowd

Get used to this dream, it is very common among pregnant women and new mothers. Leaving your baby or forgetting to feed it is a very real anxiety, but don't worry about it happening in real life. Nature equips babies with a strong pair of lungs and an inescapable cry to ensure that their needs are met by their mothers. Often the baby in such dreams is really a facet of the dreamer's character – that part of each of us which is vulnerable and needs looking after. Also, becoming a mother means losing a part of yourself, though not for ever. A variation on this theme is the dream of having twins, one of whom dies from some sort of neglect.

Trying to walk a tightrope or cross a narrow bridge

Dreams involving narrow passageways, bridges, tightropes or paths of any kind, are very usual during times of great change and upheaval. Pregnancy can be viewed as a sort of bridge between one way of being and another. If the journey seems perilous it could be a message from your unconscious saying you need more support from those around you. If you are travelling down a dark passageway, this may be a reflection of your anxiety about the unknown. Ask yourself which areas of your life need some light shed on them at this time.

Exposing your heavily pregnant belly to someone

This is a great dream but one which some women awake from feeling embarrassed. Remember, it's not literal, it's a metaphor. In some traditional tribes warriors expose and slap their bellies as a sign of power. Pregnant women are a symbol of life. They are very powerful creatures with great physical presence. Showing your belly to the world is a way of saying, this is me; I am here; I won't be ignored. In such dreams the reactions of the people around you are often quite telling. They may illustrate your own feelings of ambivalence, disgust, or sheer joy towards your body and your self.

Killing your mother/your mother dying

Although disturbing, this is a very symbolic dream indicating your changing role in the family. You are moving from daughter to mother.

When you become a mother your own mother's role 'dies' and evolves into that of a grandmother. You may be feeling some sympathy with her as she struggles to take on a new role and the dream may indicate a kind of rebirth for you both. Equally, you may have the kind of mother who likes to take over and the dream is telling you that it is time that her inappropriate behaviour 'died' down. How you interpret such a dream depends very much on your relationship with your mother.

The best advice when tackling a dream is to keep an open mind. Often people who try to decipher dreams in a rational way find themselves totally frustrated because they can't make 'sense' of the images before them. This is because dreams don't come from the a part of us which is sensible and logical. They come from the part of us which is creative, the place where wisdom lives. Remember that while dreams in pregnancy are often about everyday things, the meaning is rarely obvious. Even if you dream about a familiar situation, the chances are your dream is trying to communicate something new to you. Staying open to that aspect of dreamwork is challenging, but rewarding since it can bring new insight.

EVERYTHING IN MODERATION – EVEN AWARENESS

Aiming for a high level of consciousness every minute of every day is likely to raise your stress levels. We need periods of unconsciousness to balance periods of awareness, in the same way that we need periods of rest to balance periods of activity.

Discovering your spirituality is a process. It can't be achieved over the duration of a pregnancy any more than it can over the duration of a weekend workshop. All any of us can hope for is to take little steps along the way, aware that our needs in this department will change according to our age, experience and where we are in our lives at this particular time.

Exploring spirituality does not demand any special tools or settings. The repetitive vocal patterns of Buddhist chants are no more hypnotic than the click, clack of knitting needles in a quiet room. Insights gained while lying in the bath, digging the garden or washing the dishes are every bit as legitimate and profound as those gained in deep meditation in a dark room scented with sandalwood and patchouli. Sometimes they are more so, since they will have occurred in the context of your day-to-day life.

Being pregnant will expand your horizons in all sorts of directions. At times it can seem an impossible task to keep up with the demands which such changes place upon you. Give yourself a break, and remember that it's not whether you doggedly pursue consciousness, spirituality and insight, but whether you are open to them when they come which matters more.

CHAPTER 5

CHANGING RELATIONSHIPS

Things will change. Pregnancy – particularly for the first time – signals the turning of life's wheel. Each of us lives on many levels at once and is involved in many different kinds of relationships: to ourselves, to our intimate partners, to our families, friends and colleagues, to our communities and to our Gods.

The birth of a baby, a dramatic enough event in its own right, is like a drop into a still pool. It sends out ripples of change in every direction. Nobody remains untouched by the birth of a child; lovers become parents, daughter becomes mother, mother becomes grandmother, husband becomes father, sister becomes aunt, nephews and nieces become cousins and close friends become adopted aunts, uncles and sometimes godparents. Some welcome the change in roles and responsibilities, others find the adjustment more difficult.

Other relationships also undergo a transformation during this time. Many women, once pregnant, feel the need to stay closer to the community in which they live. This can sometimes be a surprising experience, since the community which seemed adequate in your non-pregnant state may seem suddenly hostile now that you are a mother.

You may, for instance, look around and ask yourself: are there places to sit down when you are tired? Can you breastfeed in your usual shops? Is there somewhere to buy or eat fresh food? Is there somewhere to meet other mothers who share your world view? What is the community's attitude towards lone mothers? Is there support in the form of doulas or birth sisters? What are the facilities for care before, during and after birth? What about childcare? The community is an important source of support for soon-to-be and new parents. Many a pregnant woman has looked around only to find that hers is sorely lacking. The resulting feelings of abandonment can sometimes be quite profound.

In addition, your relationship to God, or whatever higher being you acknowledge, as well as to the creative power of the universe and to Nature, will also be challenged. You may feel an increased interest in the religious beliefs of your family, adapting them to your needs or abandoning them altogether.

In more traditional cultures birth is a social event celebrated by the whole community. Among the Navajo Indians of North America, when a mother goes into labour, the whole tribe gathers around to eat a meal and enjoy the show.

Now is the time to begin to acknowledge that life and death are not wholly within human control. For some, the realization that being born is about as safe as life gets is comforting. It makes them feel a part of something bigger and more divine than mundane human existence. For others, it is a terrifying notion which makes them feel small and insignificant. Our reactions to the process of pregnancy and birth, how we interpret and act upon concepts such as 'safety' and 'risk', often stem from such realizations.

Of all your relationships, however, it may be the ones closest to home which need the most care and attention.

As a woman, your relationship to yourself will have begun to change almost from the moment you knew you were pregnant. It takes a mighty amount of psychological and emotional adjustment to take on board the idea that there is another human life growing inside your body. You may experience a new sort of commitment to yourself which may be expressed through changing your diet and cutting down or cutting out cigarettes and alcohol. You may be taking regular exercise and balancing this with rest and recreation. You may also be more aware now of the intuitive side of your nature and your capacity for emotional highs as well as lows. For the first time your desire to stay true to yourself may clash with the reality of living in a world which encourages conformity.

In the West we like to think that we thrive on change, but in reality we are not very adaptable. Change is welcomed only if it is directed at the most superficial layers of our lives; thus we seek and celebrate changes in our hairstyles, clothes, homes and cars. But when the impetus comes to change who we are and how we function at the very deepest levels, we sometimes struggle. Many people associate change with a worsening of their situation – and occasionally this is true. But change can also be positive. Certainly the dynamics of your closest relationships will often alter dramatically, and the more dependent the relationship pre-pregnancy, the greater the sense of loss and resentment will be when it is compelled to change. Some may break under the strain, but this is not inevitable – much can be done to ensure that the changes of pregnancy, birth and parenthood support rather than undermine who we are.

INTO THE MYSTERY

Both men and women experience a steep learning curve once a baby is on the way but, on the whole, women have more practical resources (in the form of books and antenatal courses) to help them cope. For this and other reasons there is often what social scientists refer to as a 'his and hers pregnancy' going on in the same household, with neither party feeling as if their feelings count or are totally understood.

A man whose partner is pregnant is meeting two mysteries at once: the mystery of medicine and the mystery of a woman's body. Although it may seem strange to talk about medicine as a kind of mysticism, observation of what goes on in most hospitals and antenatal clinics reveals that they rely on ritual, routine and the illusion of 'mysterious' power, in much the same way ancient shamans did.

These medical mysteries can be unbelievably frustrating. Medical practitioners seem to excel at talking endlessly while avoiding any meaningful kind of communication. 'Patients' are sometimes talked down to, led to believe that the birth process is too complex for anyone other than a doctor to understand, and encouraged to place their faith in medical magic. A man may enter the system wanting to become informed and protect his partner, but come out feeling the need of some protection himself!

'A man should never get angry at his wife while she is pregnant, for his raised voice turns seven times in her vagina and reaches the child.'
WEST AFRICAN SAYING

Although it is rarely acknowledged, expectant fathers are as much victims of cultural and medical stereotyping as women are. Many doctors and midwives have seriously fixed ideas about men's place in the scheme of things. Often their involvement in antenatal appointments, in classes and during labour is merely tolerated, rather than openly welcomed. Many men report that hospital staff treat them as if they are in the way.

TV and films also have a lot to answer for in helping to shape our perception of fathers. The images we see of men during labour teach us that a man's role is to be either comical or cowardly, controlled or controlling.

Is it any wonder so many men have mixed feelings about being involved in the experience of pregnancy and birth? In the absence of any helpful preparation for this role during adolescence, most rely on what they have heard from other men, what they have read, the signals they are receiving from medical staff and, of course, what they have seen in the media to provide a role for them. It must scare them to death.

Men and women also have a different perception of time during pregnancy. Because the baby is inside her, a woman feels the passing of time with greater urgency, punctuated as it is by bodily changes and the increasingly strong kicks of her child. A pregnant woman is emotionally and physically pregnant every second of every day. She cannot escape the experience. A man, however, may only begin to think about the pregnancy and interact with it as the baby begins to move or after attending a first scan. When he's not with his pregnant partner, a man may not think about it at all. It is not unusual for a man to feel that he has all the time in the world to come to terms with parenthood until the last few weeks of pregnancy, when he suddenly panics and realizes he hasn't read a relevant book or been to a single antenatal class.

Even this temporary divide is enough to create resentment within a relationship. For those women who are not happy being pregnant, and for those who just occasionally feel trapped, the fact that their man can escape the experience can cause powerful resentment. He may not even intend to escape, he may simply be responding to the demands of his work, but the fact that he is not living the pregnancy with the same minute-by-minute intensity is very threatening.

When it comes to feelings, the new intensity which motivates a woman during pregnancy can also be difficult to relate to and can make a man feel more ignorant. While some men respond to this feeling by wanting to know everything that goes on at the clinic and devouring all the books their wives are reading, others react in a more defensive way. Unhappy about their state of ignorance these men will, when asked, come out with statements like, 'Well it's all common sense, isn't it?', or 'You've got it all under control, what do you need my opinion for?', or 'I'm just going to take it as it comes.'

This can be terribly frustrating for a woman who desperately wants her partner to bring the same sort of intelligence, commitment and sensitivity that he would to his job, to being adequately prepared for the reality of birth and parenting their soon-to-be-born child. For a man, admitting that he doesn't know something can be very difficult. It puts him in an inferior position to his partner at a time when he is already feeling unsure of himself. This is why the sense of a shared journey is so important from the beginning.

Happily, no relationship will be in this state all the time. The majority of couples experience a fluid state where the relationship changes from day to day. You may both need to be more sensitive to these changes in order to make progress. Learn to pick the best moments in which to talk things through. Be aware that things change and although you may both be feeling a sense of shock and abandonment during the first few months, it may not last much further into the pregnancy. If your partner has been playing 'catch up' he may feel a little more a part of things during the middle months, when he can also feel the baby move. Don't lose faith in the fact that some men are quietly impressed by a woman's

The Ga women of Africa believe that they can transfer any pregnancy-related illness to their partners. To do this they step over their partner's sleeping bodies during the night so that he takes on their discomforts for the duration of the pregnancy. It seems to work. The Ga women have a reputation for being hale and hearty when pregnant, while the men often report being sickly.

ability to create another human being. Many take pride in their partner's increasingly obvious pregnancy as a symbol of their own involvement and their own fertility.

If the lines of communication are good in your relationship, it is possible to meet (maybe even defeat) the inevitable anxieties which new parenthood brings into a relationship, and the miracle taking place in your body can become a shared experience.

Talk About It Now

Long before the antenatal classes start it is a good idea to establish basic information together. Shared parenting doesn't just evolve magically. When all is said and done the most important common ground you may have consists of your views on parenthood and divisions of labour.

The value of this can become quickly apparent. For example, if a woman has a traditional view of parenting and her partner is a 'new man' type, there is bound to be friction. Negotiating these boundaries early, while there are fewer demands on your time and energy, can help avoid conflict later on. Communication about values, hopes and beliefs and the practicalities of life with a new baby, by the way, is just as important with second and subsequent babies as it is with a first-born.

Have you considered:
• Why do you want to be parents? Or if this is not your first baby, why are you having another child?
• What kind of parents do you each want to be? Life can be tough if you have conflicting ideas about traditional versus modern parenting styles.
• Parental love is expressed, particularly in the early days, through a series of tasks – feeding, changing, comforting, playing and cleaning – which must be done. Who will do these?
• The impact of a new baby on your finances? New parenthood can often mean going into debt. Where are you prepared to economize?
• Where will the money come from? Who should work and who should stay at home?
• What about childcare? What are your needs and hopes? What sort of childcare best meets these? What is available in your area?

• Is the house big enough? Do you need to move? Would moving mean more stress than living in a small space?

• Housework – who is going to do what and when – and to what level of competence? It can be unbelievably frustrating to turn a household job over to someone only to find that they have done a poor or half-hearted job.

• Who will have the final say in an argument over, for instance, a purchasing decision? Don't get so caught up in the idea of democracy that you end up being unable to make a choice.

• What are your views about your child's schooling? About healthcare? Again, differing belief systems can cause arguments over matters we take for granted, such as vaccinations and discipline.

• Other children – how will each of your responsibilities to them change with the arrival of another child?

This is only a small selection of the kinds of things which can sneak up on you and cause conflict. Don't be too worried if you can't resolve every issue immediately. Keeping the lines of communication open is the most important thing. Even if you have to revise some of your ideas after the baby arrives, talking about them beforehand shows commitment and can help to defuse potentially stressful situations afterwards.

HIS PREGNANCY

Men experience their own ups and downs during pregnancy. Over the years social scientists have identified three stages – action, doubt and couvade – which men go through during their partners' pregnancy. Interestingly, these roughly correspond to the three trimesters of pregnancy.

Stage 1 – Action The action phase is mostly about making plans. It usually revolves around lifestyle changes and working out a strategy for taking time off work after the baby arrives. Some women find this phase comforting, even though their partner's attention may be on something other than them. Primarily this is because the action phase corresponds to a time when the woman herself may be feeling sick and tired and unable to carry on as usual. Her partner's 'action' provides the necessary reassurance that things will go on as normal for a while.

Stage 2 – Doubt Action, however, is soon replaced by doubt – about himself, about his partner, and about the baby. This is a time when men begin to worry about a wide variety of things including money, work, the health of their child, the birth, their ability to be 'good' fathers, feelings of ignorance and foolishness and changes in their relationship with the woman they love, especially with regard to 'being left out' and 'playing second fiddle to the baby'.

Men also have to come to terms with their changing roles. Being a pregnant father brings up doubts, insecurities and worries. It brings back childhood memories, questions about their relationships with their own fathers (and mothers). If the woman is also feeling insecure, she may unwittingly fall back on that old cultural stereotype of the man being strong and silent while she is allowed more or less full rein of her emotions. This leaves the man with even fewer outlets to express his true feelings.

Unfortunately these overwhelming feelings of doubt roughly correspond to the time when most women are getting into their stride and beginning to feel more confident. With morning sickness behind them and the baby's first movements being detected, this is a period when most women really begin to enjoy pregnancy.

Stage 3 – Couvade Couvade is an old-fashioned term for the time when a man begins to experience the same emotional upheaval and physical pains as a woman. Traditionally it referred only to the period during labour, but more recently the definition has widened to include late pregnancy as well. This is the time when some men become unnervingly interested in their pets or deeply emotional about sports activities and news reports. They may suddenly become fitness fanatics or decide to start that novel or screenplay they've been brooding over for years. In traditional tribes, men under the influence of couvade would feel the same aches and pains as their labouring womenfolk. During labour, it is said that their experience of the same intense pains drew evil spirits away from the actual birth.

As many as seven out of every ten men get mysterious pains – backaches, stomach aches, nausea, constipation, cravings and aversions to foods – when their partners are pregnant. As long as it doesn't detract attention from the woman, couvade can be seen in an admirable light – a way of trying to empathize with the woman's experience, to make a connection with his child and as a public declaration of paternity and responsibility.

Are You Supportable?

Some women can, without intending to, exclude their partners from what they are going through, physically and emotionally. When this happens both partners can become further isolated in their own lonely experience of pregnancy. The reasons why women might do this are complex. In part it may be that in all other areas of life men are powerful creatures who like to take control. Some women may feel that to allow a man too much involvement in the process of pregnancy and birth would be to invite him to take over completely, and certainly some men do react in this way. But not all men want to be in control. Many are genuinely fascinated by and admiring of the changes which occur in their wives' bodies and simply want to share the experience as best they can.

It can also be hard for a strong woman to let herself go into the experience of pregnancy which, by its very nature, puts her in a dependent position. But once you are pregnant it can be very draining to have to take on all the battles on the home front by yourself. Even if this has been your pattern before, now is the time to let your man do some of the battling for you. Don't argue with the plumber or the gas company, don't wait in huge queues at the post office or drag heavy groceries back from the market on your own. And don't become isolated in your dealings with people at hospitals and clinics. Providing you and your partner have discussed fully what you want out of the birth and he is prepared to support you – and providing he can get the time off – it can be a great comfort to have him with you at antenatal appointments.

Some competent women resist turning to their partner for support and justify this by saying 'he doesn't have a clue' about what their needs are. While it can help to vent your frustrations to a sympathetic friend, it is not any more noble to be a 'victim' in your relationship than it is to be a victim of medical meddling. A better alternative is to help him to help you. Find strategies which ensure that your partner hears you and can meet your needs.

For instance, many women enjoy and derive great benefit from a good massage, particularly later in pregnancy. However, not all men are confident in their skills as a masseur. If you go to a reflexologist or for a shiatsu massage during pregnancy, or if you see an osteopath or an aromatherapist, why not consider having your partner come along to a few 'teaching' sessions? Even if you don't go to this kind of therapist regularly, consider contacting a local practitioner who you know works with pregnant women and asking him or her to help advise your partner on how and where to massage you. Your partner may resist the idea at first, but remind him that he will be acquiring a skill which will inspire confidence and come in very handy, again and again, over the course of your life together.

Although men and women don't always realize it, pregnancy is a time when a woman needs her partner more than ever. It is a time when many women have a desire to be taken care of in the same competent way in which they have been taking care of their men, often for years. While some men lose interest, it is a time when the majority would love to be a part of it all if only they knew how.

It is unreasonable, however, to assume that your partner will anticipate and fulfil your every need. Therefore, along with everything else, you may need to learn how to ask for what you want without nagging, giving a long list of reasons why it should be done or using emotional blackmail. Even though your husband loves you he probably can't read your mind. There may even be times during pregnancy when, like the proverbial toddler, you don't know what you want, but you want it now!

Rules for supporters and the supported are simple:
- Giving support does not mean taking away responsibility. Giving

support is often a passive act. It does not involve doing for the other person but loving them, listening to them and legitimizing what they are going through. In order to support someone you have to assume they have achieved a level of competence and wisdom in what they are doing. Men who are used to being in charge, should be encouraged to think of being supportive as a dance. Although one partner is obliged to follow the other's lead, the end result is two bodies and minds working as one.

• Accepting support is not the same as being helpless. It is entirely possible to accept support without becoming dependent and weak. Indeed, it can sometimes take a high level of competence and strength of character to acknowledge the need for support. Especially when you are heavily pregnant, you will need help with everyday activities such as lifting things or getting in and out of the car, vacuuming the stairs or cleaning the bath. Now is the time to contemplate the subtle differences between independence and interdependence and try to differentiate between help – where someone may take over all or part of your duties and chores – and support – where energy is directed into helping you navigate your journey yourself.

To be supportable you must understand the difference.

CHANGING SEXUALITY

A 'good' sexual relationship is the product of patience, love, understanding and practice. It can't be built in a day or a night. When the honeymoon period is over the hard work begins and most couples, pregnant or otherwise, will experience times when for one reason or another there is a disruption in the rhythm of their sexual lives. Because most babies are born to younger women in relatively new relationships, it is likely that the first time a couple experience this kind of disruption is when the woman is pregnant.

Older couples, or those who have been together longer, will already know that as a relationship develops, disruption, lack of interest and sexual dysfunction can strike either partner at any time. In a committed relationship you learn to roll with it, recognizing that sometimes sex is good and sometimes it is bad; sometimes it's dutiful and other times it's like a million bright fireworks. But if this is the first time a sexual disagreement has hit your relationship it can come as quite a shock, and the usual response is to begin to point the finger of blame – at each other and at the baby.

During pregnancy you may experience more pronounced emotional highs and lows in your relationship. There can be increased closeness and sharing, but also increased conflicts and feelings of isolation. Often these feelings get acted out in the bedroom and mismatched levels of sexual desire are one of the most common areas of conflict during pregnancy and after birth.

There is no consensus even among traditional cultures about sex during pregnancy. The Truk women in Micronesia believe that sex during pregnancy can cause miscarriages, or give the child a birthmark or a harelip. But according to the Pacific Trobriand islanders, intercourse provides an important source of nourishment for the child.

It would be wrong, however, to paint a picture of changing sexuality that is primarily focused on a reduction in activity. And it would also be wrong to say that it is always women who don't want to have sex. For some couples, without the worries about contraception, sex becomes fun, relaxing and rejuvenating. A significant proportion of women experience a greatly increased need for and enjoyment in sex. The greater amount of blood circulating around their genital area and breasts means that these areas are more sensitive and more easily aroused.

In some couples it is the man, alarmed by his partner's changing body, by the weight of his new responsibilities, by feelings of envy towards his wife's experience of pregnancy, who halts or restricts sexual activity.

Most couples, however, fall somewhere in between, with their sexual desires more or less in tune some of the time, out of tune some of the time, and in a not unpleasant neutral state the rest of the time.

When mismatches do occur, lack of love or lack of caring is rarely the problem. More often it is the inability, due to fear or lack of emotional resources, to understand what is important to the other person and to acknowledge it, even if it is different from what you want and need.

There is also the problem of not knowing how to ask for what you want. Sex, like money, is something which many of us find very difficult to talk about. In relationships, women and men therefore often fall prey to the romantic fantasy that their other half should simply 'know'. This ignores the fact that the partner may be shy, emotionally inarticulate or simply too exhausted by the rigours of new parenthood to 'know' any more. If problems between you and your partner seem too difficult to sort out, now may be a good time to consider seeking the help of a couples counsellor. Often having a safe space, away from home, to talk about difficulties can be a substantial step in the direction of a solution.

Although it sounds like a cliché, now is really the time to start discussing and exploring other ways of giving pleasure and communicating love and attraction. Touching, massage, kissing and foot and back rubs will all help to maintain an intimate link between the two of you.

Now is also the time to think quality instead of quantity. Once you allow the frequency, or lack of it, of your lovemaking to become an issue it can be very hard to let the subject drop. Communication is the key, since it can reassure you both that there is still love. Communication also fosters creativity. By talking it through you may be able to share ideas about how best to keep intimacy alive at times when for whatever reason intercourse is not possible. You can also begin to explore new lovemaking positions which enrich your love life while serving the practical need of keeping the man's weight off the woman's abdomen.

You might try not making intercourse and/or orgasm the single goal of sexual contact, even if it is for one night a week. Some couples may grumble that sex without these things is pointless, but if the alternative is no sex, hurt feelings and a continual state of impasse, isn't it worth a try? Your relationship as a couple forms the foundation of your soon-to-emerge family. Now is the time to make the foundation stronger.

YOUR OTHER CHILDREN

If there are other children in your family then there is the possibility of them feeling left out or threatened by the new baby. This does not always happen, however, and it is wise not to anticipate big problems. Instead, try to respond to whatever signals your child is giving out. If the child is very young, the idea of a new baby will seem even less real than it may to your husband. Trying to make such a child understand what is about to happen may prove frustrating for both of you.

The experience of antenatal teachers is that when birth is treated as a family event, there are rarely problems of intense sibling jealousy. The problem is that birth is now rarely treated thus. Turning it into an event which takes place in the hospital environment almost always means that other children are excluded. They associate birth with their mother being away from them, sometimes whisked away in an ambulance.

To help your other children adjust:

• *Show them you love them.* It sounds simplistic, but when the business of preparing for another child takes over, it can be easy to forget to spend some time with your other child and to say 'I love you' every day.

• *Let them know they are important.* If your other child is old enough, now may be a good time to let them have special responsibilities around the house. Doing something of value to the family makes the child feel more a part of the family. If these tasks can centre on preparing for the new baby, all the better.

• *Keep them informed.* If you are tired and cranky say so. Lashing out at a young child for not 'knowing' is pointless and can be cruel. Own up to your own feelings so your child doesn't feel that they are somehow his or her fault.

• *Let them express their own feelings.* Older siblings often feel a tremendous pressure to 'be good'. To many this means suppressing 'bad' feelings such as frustration, anger and resentment. Censoring your child's feelings closes down the lines of communication. Make a habit of this and you may wake up one morning and realize you don't know who your children are any more.

• *Remember, they value your presence.* Making time for your older child is very important – even if it means leaving the baby with a friend or relative for an hour or two. You won't know how your child is feeling or what they need unless you make this contact. If a child is feeling blue, being the centre of mum or dad's attention for a little while is often the best medicine.

There is no right or wrong time to tell your other children that you are pregnant. Some parents wait until the pregnancy has progressed past three months and the fear of miscarriage has subsided. There may be wisdom in this if your other children are very young. On the other hand miscarriage is also part of the experience of birth and some children can be remarkably insightful and understanding when it occurs. The best advice is always to follow your instincts on how best to break the news.

If your other child or children do feel jealous occasionally it's not a sign that you have failed as a parent. Sibling rivalry can happen at any time, in any family. However, by making time for your other child or children and including them from the very beginning in the experience of pregnancy and birth, you may find that feelings of jealousy are less intense.

WRITING A LETTER TO YOUR MOTHER

When you are pregnant, and for some considerable time afterwards, your relationship to your own parents will undergo some changes. The form which these changes take depends on what your relationship was like pre-pregnancy. Sometimes the relationship improves dramatically as you begin to see your parents in a new light or as equals at last. The sense of sharing a common experience is very powerful and is one which can bring you closer together. But sometimes the relationship deteriorates, a situation as sad as it is difficult to remedy.

Of all the family relations, the changing dynamic between mother and daughter is among the most difficult to negotiate during pregnancy. Many mothers greet the news that they are about to become grandmothers with mixed emotions. Becoming a grandmother means handing the reins over to someone else. It means acknowledging that your 'little girl' has grown up and is living her own life. It also means acknowledging that you are growing older.

Some potential grandmothers react to this by resisting the change. It is not unusual to find this type of woman trying to control every aspect of her daughter's pregnancy. In this type of relationship the daughter may already be well adapted to letting her mother take over.

But for many, becoming a mother signals an opportunity to carve out a life of their own design. Even if you have been a more or less compliant, 'good girl' in your mother's eyes until now, you may begin to feel a deep longing to run your own life. You may become aware of gaps in your sexual education or you may not agree with the way your mother thinks things should be handled. Such feelings can be difficult to express to your mother's face. Love, respect and sometimes fear conspire to keep you silent. Nevertheless, once they emerge, conflicting feelings about your mother need to be addressed. Some women need and genuinely benefit from the help of a therapist when embarking on this path.

A good way to begin on your own, however, is to write a letter to your mother. *This is a letter which you will not send.* Instead, it is a way to make sense of what you are feeling and give it voice. Such a letter may, eventually, provide the starting point for real conversations with your mother. Some productive topics for consideration are:

- What kind of parent was she? What would you like to do differently?
- Was her perception of the female body positive or negative?
- Was her attitude to sex open and honest? Was it secret and fearful?
- What was her own experience of being born? Of giving birth? How did it affect her beliefs?
- Her spirituality – is it the same as yours or different?
- Does she accept you as a competent adult?
- Breastfeeding – did she or didn't she? How do you feel about it either way?
- Child abuse – was she the abuser? Did she stand passively by while you were abused by someone else?
- Was she able to show affection? Did you feel loved?
- When she expressed anger, was it appropriate and 'clean' or did anger mix with blame to hurt everyone else in the family? Was anger repressed?

The chances are your style of parenting will be eclectic, taking the best from what you had as a child and mixing it with new elements acquired along your own life path. Writing it out is a good way of getting your own feelings in perspective.

It also becomes a powerful tool for understanding the women who raised us, and letting go of some of our resentments and feelings of blame. Remembering how you felt as a child brings you one step closer to understanding your own child. Allowing anger and resentment to fall away clears the way for you to become the parent you want to be, instead of simply reacting to your own childhood.

CHAPTER 6

A LABOUR OF LOVE

Ninety per cent of women will become mothers at some stage in their lives and each of them will have to confront the issue of how to give birth in their own way. When thinking ahead to labour, however, few are encouraged to try to make the experience an expression of who they are and what they believe. Instead, most women's attention is directed towards choosing levels of pain relief and ways to reduce the time spent in labour.

Today's hospitals practise what is known as active management of labour, enforcing strict rules about how long labour will be 'allowed' to last. Active management is mostly a bureaucratic exercise, the aim of which is to process as many women as possible through the hospital system in the shortest possible space of time. It has never been shown to improve the safety of birth and many women have expressed negative feelings about its impact after the event. Research over the last 20 years since its implementation tells us what women intuitively suspect: active management does not reduce pain or significantly shorten the length of labour.

Under active management a woman's waters will be broken shortly after arrival at hospital and her labour induced or hastened. If she doesn't give birth to her child within the given time limit (usually within 24 hours for a first child and 12 hours for a second and subsequent babies) some action – either an episiotomy, forceps, ventouse or an 'emergency' caesarean – will be taken to complete the job for her. Because speeding up labour can make it more painful, the actively managed woman may be given pain-relieving drugs which may include gas and air (Entonox), pethidine and epidural anaesthesia, often in combination and all in the space of a few hours to 'help' her cope. Each of these interventions alters the normal experience of labour and is capable of producing a negative impact on the well-being of the mother and her baby (*see* table overleaf).

Labour-Saving Devices

Device	Advantages	Disadvantages
ARM (Artificial Rupture of the Membranes) Breaking open the protective sac of water which surrounds the baby in the womb	• There are no advantages to its routine use. However, in a lengthy, *established* labour ARM may help move things along	• Disrupts the natural course of labour • Increases the risk of cord prolapse, which deprives the baby of oxygen • The baby's heart rate can drop after it is done • Can increase the pain of labour • Increases the risk of infection • The procedure is painful • It doesn't always work • Can cause breathing difficulties in the baby
Synthetic hormones An oxytocin drip or prostaglandin pessaries used to induce or speed up labour	• There are no advantages to routine use, though it can be useful to stimulate labour for a woman whose baby has died *in utero*	• Can produce unmanageably strong contractions, particularly when on a continuous drip or when repeated pessaries are used • Requires continuous fetal monitoring • Reduced mobility for the mother • Increases risk of an unnecessary caesarean • Can cause fetal distress • Increases the risk of post-partum haemorrhage, especially for those with caesarean scars • May cause breathing difficulties in the baby • Can cause neonatal jaundice
Intermittent monitoring Monitoring the baby's heartbeat with a Pinard, stethoscope or hand-held sonic aid	• Decreases the likelihood of a false diagnosis of fetal distress • Less invasive than continual monitoring • Can be done in any position, even under water • Increases the amount of personal attention a labouring woman gets	• There are no disadvantages for a healthy mother and baby. However, a sonic aid is an ultrasonic device which the mother may wish to avoid
EFM (Electronic Fetal Monitoring) Ultrasonic device, usually a belt, used to monitor the fetal heartbeat and sometimes the strength of the mother's contractions	• Can be reassuring, especially if the baby is at risk • Necessary once there have been interventions such as induction	• Reduced mobility can increase fetal distress • Belts can be uncomfortable • Exposes your baby to further ultrasound • Raises the risk of false diagnosis of fetal distress • Hospital staff not always adequately trained to use the machine • Has become substitute for personal care and professional judgement
Fetal scalp electrode An ultrasonic monitor which is screwed into the baby's scalp	• Can give a more accurate assessment of the baby's well-being than an external monitor	• Painful for the baby • Can cause the baby's heart rate to drop • Increases the risk of infection after birth • Leaves a scar on the baby
Forceps or Ventouse Steel blades (forceps) or a suction device (ventouse) applied to the baby's head and used to extract it from the womb. Ventouse will generally cause less trauma to the baby's head than forceps	• An aid to delivery in cases of fetal distress • If mother's uterus is over-stimulated by synthetic hormones often the only way, bar a caesarean, to get the baby out • Can sometimes be used to correct the baby's position to make birth more straightforward	• Often used to bring labour to a quick, but artificial, end • Both types of extraction can be painful and require an episiotomy • Painful for the baby • Lack of experience in your practitioner may result in unnecessary damage to your internal organs or to your baby's head • Many women feel a sense of failure after this type of delivery

Caesarean section

The baby is removed through an incision made through the lower abdomen and uterus

- Safe delivery of the baby in cases of placenta praevia
- Appropriate for those with fulminating pre-eclampsia, unstable heart conditions or kidney disease
- Can be performed quickly in cases of fetal distress
- A simple operation for your doctor to perform

- It is major abdominal surgery
- Nearly half of all operations are unnecessary
- The mother is 4 to 6 times more likely to die than those giving birth vaginally
- Babies are often born prematurely
- Difficult to establish breastfeeding afterwards
- Reduces future fertility
- Future pregnancies have an increased risk of placenta accretia where the placenta becomes intractably imbedded in the womb, increasing risk of serious post-partum haemorrhage
- Higher rate of depression for mothers
- Risk of post-surgical infection – caesarean mothers take more antibiotics than others
- Caesarean mothers take more painkillers
- Impact on future births – many women are denied the opportunity to give birth vaginally
- Increases the rate of breathing difficulties in babies

Gas and Air

Mild pain relief. Inhaled mixture of nitrous oxide and oxygen, also known as Entonox

- Takes the edge off the pain
- Most useful during transition

- Effect lasts only 60 seconds
- Nausea and dizziness are a common side effect
- Alters your state of consciousness but does not take the pain away
- Used during the second stage can interfere with bearing-down efforts
- Increases the risk of subsequent drug addiction in babies when used in large doses

Pethidine

Morphine derivative given by injection

- In very small doses a useful uterine muscle relaxant
- May be useful in small doses if taken before the mother reaches 7cm dilation

- Does not take the pain away
- Women report loss of confidence and a feeling of hopelessness as a side effect
- Slows mother's breathing down so less oxygen to the baby
- Linked to breathing problems in the baby
- Nausea is common
- Increased risk of drug addiction for the child later in life

Epidural

Cocaine derivative injected into the area around the spine

- Eliminates all sensation of pain
- Mother will be awake during a caesarean operation
- Post-operative pain relief
- A well-timed epidural can be left to wear off so that the mother can push the baby out herself

- Increased risk of unnecessary caesarean operations
- In 10 to 33 per cent of cases the epidural fails to work
- Slackens pelvic-floor muscles and so prolongs labour
- Increases the risk of dystocia – the baby getting stuck in the birth canal
- Increases the risk of unnecessary forceps and ventouse deliveries
- Higher rates of episiotomy
- Mother will be lying down, often in one position for a long period of time, increasing the risk of fetal distress
- Long-term backache is a common side effect
- Long-term headaches are also reported
- The baby may be born with a high temperature which may lead to the administration of unnecessary antibiotics
- More breathing difficulties for the baby
- The baby may be more 'fussy' than others and have difficulty breastfeeding

In recent years, actively managed birth, which as many as 70 per cent of women will experience to a greater or lesser degree, has become synonymous with 'normal' birth, even though the two are clearly not the same. It is *actively managed* birth, not *normal* birth, which the majority of women have come to fear.

It is never too early to start thinking about your priorities for labour. Although it lasts only a relative few hours, the way a woman experiences labour can affect her life in profound and unexpected ways. You will never forget your birth experience and you can't go back and do it again if things go wrong. Studies into women's attitudes towards labour show that those who know what they want are the ones most likely to get it. They are also the women who are most likely to report feelings of satisfaction with the process of birth, *whatever the outcome*. Conversely, women who remain undecided or who allow others to take over, are the ones who feel the most disempowered by the experience.

In sorting out her priorities for labour, each woman should be encouraged to ask herself some relevant questions: Does labour really need to be managed? Is it just a redundant step between being pregnant and holding a baby in your arms? Is it a process which has outlived its evolutionary usefulness? Is birth only safe in retrospect? Would the whole process of becoming a parent be a lot more satisfying if we could do away with labour altogether? Can pain ever be positive? How she answers these questions will, to a large extent, provide the basis for her choices about labour.

IS LABOUR JUST A PAIN?

It has come to a sad and rather frightening state of affairs when an alternative approach to birth requires, first and foremost, a redefinition of labour as a normal bodily function.

The experience of labour doesn't always feel normal, however, because it is often accompanied by numerous medical interventions. And while even a relatively straightforward birth can at times be painful and emotionally overwhelming, given the right conditions it can also be powerful, joyous, funny, loving and gentle. It is our preoccupation with labour as a lot of unnecessary pain (and the things which we do to try to avoid that pain), which turns a rich and varied moment in a woman's life into a one-dimensional experience.

Because the pain of birth is a universal experience, assume for a moment that it is pain, not painlessness, which is normal. Since nature rarely does anything without a purpose, it's worth asking what the purpose of pain in labour might be. There appear to be two answers. Physiologically, a woman needs to know when she is in labour. She needs to know how

Malaysian midwives feel a woman's feet to tell them if labour is imminent. If the big toe is cold, it means that the blood has started to leave her extremities and travel to the uterus. If the ankle is cold as well it means that birth is imminent. They believe that as the blood is drawn to the uterus the environment in the womb gets hotter and the baby doesn't like it and wants to come out.

far along she is and whether the birth of her baby is imminent. The different types and levels of pain which a woman feels at different stages of labour provide this information.

Psychologically, working with or submitting to the power of labour offers an opportunity for self-discovery which is unique to women. Those who have experienced labour without the usual pain-relieving drugs may go through a powerful psychological transition which women who have chosen to eliminate the pain may not experience.

Certainly there is no evidence that women's levels of satisfaction with birth are linked to the absence of pain. In fact for some, taking away the pain of birth may significantly diminish its quality and significance. Interestingly, the women most likely to express dissatisfaction with birth are those who have had epidurals and had no sensation of pain at all.

Levels of pain in labour are not predestined and can rise and fall according to the kind of social support a mother has, whether she feels safe in her place of birth, her own level of fear about the birth process, what position her body is in, the way the baby is lying and what interventions, if any, she has had. What is more, in a normal labour the level of pain builds gradually, allowing the mother time to adjust physically and psychologically. But how many labours today are normal?

It is also important to make a distinction between the woman who chooses and the woman who is unable to refuse. Some women may choose narcotic pain relief when all other reasonable methods have failed or because of its occasionally medicinal effect (for instance, pethidine can be an effective muscle relaxant and the epidural can lower blood pressure). Others, for instance the mother who is overcome by fear or whose labour has been induced or who has been rendered immobile by continuous monitoring and a drip, may be in such pain that she is in no position to refuse extreme forms of pain relief. Under such circumstances, drugs do become 'necessary'.

Nevertheless, after all the arguments are put on the table, pain is usually the one thing (next to tearing or episiotomy) that women fear most. In response to women's confusion and fear a number of different drugs – analgesics, tranquillizers and anaesthetics – have been concocted to relieve the pain of birth. Some are more effective than others and, ironically, the more effective the drug is at relieving the mother's pain, the greater number of adverse effects it has on her baby.

Medical research has also turned up an interesting side note about why so many doctors and midwives are so enthusiastic about the use of pain-relieving drugs in labour: women who have epidurals are quieter and less demanding. For many medical practitioners the epidural is the pain reliever of choice, because by blocking out any sensation of pain it maintains a sense of calm and quiet on the labour ward. Unlike pethidine, which alters a woman's state of consciousness, a woman who has an epidural remains alert. This, of course, brings up an uncomfortable question: for whom are such forms of pain relief the most beneficial?

The information which women receive about the pros and cons of narcotic pain relief is often misleading. Unfortunately many doctors and midwives are gravely misinformed about the side-effects of routine pain relief. The most common misconception is that pain-relieving drugs, especially the epidural, do not cross the placenta. *All* drugs cross the placenta, though some appear to do less damage than others.

When considering the use of pain-relieving drugs, we tend to focus on the immediate future, both in terms of benefit and adverse effects.

However, studies in Sweden on the long-term effects for babies whose mothers used drugs such as pethidine and Entonox during labour make disturbing reading. These show a link between drug use in labour and drug addiction in later life due to what is known as imprinting – a memory etched into the mind during a short, sensitive period leading to specific behaviours in adult life.

Labour involves a certain amount of stress for a baby. If during this important time drugs, which relieve that stress, enter the baby's bloodstream, the baby has received the message that this is the appropriate response to stress. While addiction itself is not the result of imprinting, the tendency to use and abuse drugs is thought to be. The greater availability and social acceptance of drugs today means that more and more young adults may respond to this unconscious imprint.

This was good-quality research which was largely ignored by the medical community and the media. It was 'bad' news; it was information which might 'worry' mothers, and it has not been adequately followed up by more studies. Although such findings represent the extreme end of the spectrum of potential side-effects of pain-relieving drugs, it opens the door for mothers to ask another important but difficult question: *what else haven't I been told about the side-effects of drugs in labour?*

Whether you view pain in labour as natural or unnatural, the fact is that all women use pain relief in labour. Their methods can range from self-help techniques such as being upright, being mobile, water, yoga, meditation, music, massage, homeopathic remedies and various breathing techniques to less invasive (though often not very effective) paraphernalia such as the TENS machine and the more powerful analgesics and anaesthetics.

The choice should be entirely yours. But be aware that 'natural' methods of pain relief are likely to be ineffective if brought in at the last minute. Sniffing lavender oil and sipping water infused with flower remedies are unlikely substantially to alter the course (or the pain) of a labour which has been medically directed from the beginning.

All women hope that labour won't be too painful. All women hope that labour won't be too long and arduous and that their bodies and their babies will emerge more or less intact. Few are let in on the best-kept secret in town – that it's not labour *per se*, but all the things which we do to manage it, which generally cause such problems in the first place.

A SAFE PLACE TO GIVE BIRTH

It is the natural inclination of every pregnant woman to want to give birth in a place where she feels safe.

Wherever a mother chooses to give birth, and however she chooses to give birth, she will be motivated by a desire to protect herself and her baby from harm. Although the woman who chooses a home birth and the woman who chooses an elective caesarean before term are often seen as opposites they are, in reality, motivated by the same desires for safety. And although they have come to different conclusions, they may both have gone through a process of research, consultation and reflection in order to reach that decision.

The difference between women who choose normal birth and those who choose the high-tech route isn't where they end up, it's where they begin. It's in their level of faith in themselves, how comfortable they are with their bodies, their family history, their experience of birth and the amount of support they have around them from family and friends.

A woman who is confident, body-aware and well-supported will find it much easier to challenge the medical management of pregnancy and birth. On the other hand, a woman (no matter how competent she appears superficially) who is afraid, who views her body as the enemy, who believes that birth is only safe in retrospect or who was left unsupported through a previous bad birth experience, will find that the medical view enthusiastically supports everything she has come to believe about herself.

Although doctors still advise that hospitals are the safest place for all labouring women, there is very little evidence to support this view. The issue of the relative safety of different birth venues has been thoroughly researched by many people over many years. Without exception, such studies show that the claims for the superior safety of hospitals are, at best, inflated and at worst out-and-out deception.

The vast majority of women are directed into the hospital system,

Being Overdue

An estimated due date, or EDD, is just that – an estimate. Try not to place too much significance on it, since fewer than 10 per cent of babies come on the day predicted by the EDD. Instead, try to think in terms of a range of dates on which your baby might come. Doing this will defuse any anxiety about being overdue and protect you from the often unnecessary step of being induced 'just-in-case'.

Consider this as well. Although we tend to think of the mother's body as the instigator of labour, this is not really true. It is largely the baby's readiness to be born which signals the chemical changes in the mother's body which begin the process of labour. However, certain emotional factors can also influence when labour starts.

Every pregnant woman has heard stories about those who exhibit 'nesting' behaviour just before labour begins. Such behaviour may take the form of an irresistible urge to cook, clean the house, reorganize the closet, sort socks or mend clothes.

Emotional housekeeping is also part of necessary 'nesting'. Often women who go past their due dates report that, as soon as they allow themselves to face up to whatever has been bothering them – it could be a fear of impending motherhood, or doubts about whether they could cope with birth, or an even bigger decision like a last-minute change from a hospital to a home birth – labour comes within a few hours.

When a baby is 'post-dates' the woman is bombarded with other people's opinions about what she should do. This is the complete opposite to what she needs – quiet, relaxation and contemplation. If your baby is overdue, take the phone off the hook, shut the door and listen, to yourself and your baby. Some direction or instruction from within will come and allow you to move on to the next phase, the birth of your child.

whether they need to be or not and regardless of any preferences which they might have. Many still do not appreciate that they have a choice of where their labours take place.

So many begin their pregnancies wanting as natural a pregnancy and birth as possible. Yet they choose, or are ushered into, the hospital system – a system based on science and bureaucratic efficiency – and still express surprise when the word 'natural' turns out to have no meaning in this setting.

Where you give birth will have an enormous impact on the course of your labour. For a healthy woman with a healthy baby the choice of hospital brings up some unique problems since, no matter which hospital you choose, you will still experience more routine and largely unnecessary interventions than women in any other setting, without necessarily increasing 'safety' for you or your baby. There are, however, better alternatives.

Birth at Home

Where the service is made available, a wide range of women from a variety of backgrounds tend to choose birth at home. For a woman who wants no unnecessary interventions, this is far and away the best and safest choice. When giving birth at home you may be less worried about making noises or making a 'fuss'. You will be able to eat and drink freely, you will not be restrained by monitors or drips and you can follow your inclinations about which positions feel best as your labour progresses along its natural course.

Recently a series of articles in the *British Medical Journal* concluded that, for normal women with healthy pregnancies, home birth is as safe, if not safer, than hospital birth. This finding was underlined by research from the National Birthday Trust Fund which showed that the perinatal mortality rate for hospital births was nearly five times greater than for home births. The study also showed what many others before it have – that women who give birth at home tend to be happier with the experience.

There are other benefits as well. Babies born at home tend to be bigger and healthier. Their mothers recover more quickly and are less prone to depression. Fathers also gain something. Instead of being someone who is in the way, they become full participants in their partners' labours. Also, they will not have to experience the deflating and lonely journey to an empty house after the birth of their child.

Even if you intend to give birth in hospital, you may benefit from labouring at home. In the UK the Domino scheme provides a formalized way for women to labour at home, go to hospital to deliver the baby and return home shortly afterwards. In reality, you do not need a formal scheme to do this. Even if your waters have broken, you are still safer at home where your risk of contracting infection is less and where you will not be subjected to early, unnecessary interventions. When your contractions are established and coming more frequently, that is the time to set off for the hospital.

GP or Midwifery Units

Another alternative to the big centralized hospital is the smaller GP or Midwifery unit. These small units have a consistent record of fewer interventions in labour and are staffed by midwives who work closely with GPs. Unfortunately, many of these are now under threat of closure.

In a GP unit women usually labour and give birth in the same room. It should be possible to bring personal items such as music, a bean bag, pictures, or a favourite blanket along to make the rooms, which are often very barren, more pleasant.

Women in GP units are less likely to have inductions, augmentations, forceps deliveries, epidurals, pethidine and electronic fetal monitoring (EFM). Babies fare better too. Fetal distress is twice as likely to be diagnosed in hospital and APGAR scores (the first physical assessment of the baby at one minute old) are higher in GP units.

Birthing Centres

There are very few birthing centres in the UK, unlike in the US and Australia, where their popularity is increasing. The few which do exist tend to be run by NHS or independent midwives. At a birthing centre you will have many of the facilities of a smaller GP unit and probably even less risk of interventions. Rooms will be pleasant and comfortable and there are usually extras, such as water pools to labour or give birth in.

During pregnancy you will have all your antenatal care either at home or at the centre, and some even run their own antenatal classes and postnatal support groups. The cost of a private birthing centre may be

WHAT IS A MOTHER-FRIENDLY HOSPITAL?

The phrase 'mother-friendly hospital' was coined in America and has recently begun to filter through to the UK. A mother-friendly hospital is one which does not practise routine care, but assesses the needs of each labouring woman individually.

How can you tell if your local hospital is 'mother-friendly'? Take the hospital tour, by all means, but don't be fooled by attractive decor. Many hospitals have employed decorators to make their birthing rooms look more 'homey', resulting in a profusion of rooms which are often described as being like country hotels.

Pretty wallpaper and nice curtains do not guarantee a normal birth. But they can be powerfully seductive, sometimes making mothers feel happier about the interventions they receive. If you walk into a birthing room and the bed is the most prominent piece of furniture (it's usually in the middle of the room), it is a fair indication that the pleasant surroundings are nothing more than a thin veneer to cover up fairly entrenched ideas about how and where women should give birth.

If you really want to know how 'mother-friendly' your hospital is, ask for statistics on how many caesareans they perform, how many inductions and accelerations of labour, how many forceps, ventouse and artificial ruptures of the membranes they perform, and how many home births. Your local community health council may be able to help you with such information. Be warned though, these figures often make very depressing reading.

prohibitive to some, but others reason that it is a sound investment physically, emotionally and financially in the future of the family.

YOUR BIRTH PARTNERS

Birth is an intensely personal event. Who will be with you during labour is a question which cannot be answered simply. The only certainty is that the people who surround you at this time can also have an enormous impact on the course of your labour. That is why it is important to think carefully about who you will and will not allow to share the moment with you.

Family Members

Women should feel free to choose who and how many others will be with them at the birth, but this is not always the case. In hospital there may be restrictions on who you can bring with you. Certainly you will not automatically be allowed to have your other children there. Some hospitals actively discourage the presence of 'too many' others.

Remember that hospitals are strange places, in which the expectation of disaster is just around the corner. In hospitals people naturally feel anxious and helpless and this can eventually translate into bad temper, rudeness and occasionally violent outbursts. A woman who wants a large number of her family members present in hospital should consider how well each of them might react to the tense atmosphere of the hospital and any resentment which they may encounter from staff members. The level of anxiety of those around you will have a profound effect on your labour.

Cats can be very in tune with labouring women. Many midwives and women report that if there is a cat present while the woman is labouring, the animal tends to get agitated just as she is entering transition. Many cats will spontaneously start to yowl when the women is at full dilation. As a labour support, your cat may be useful in helping you to gauge how far you are along but don't be afraid, however, to put the cat out if it starts to give you too much support!

It is usually assumed that a woman's birth partner will be her husband. In the majority of cases this may be true. But not all husbands are enthusiastic about 'being there'. Equally, not all women are thrilled about having their husbands with them. Unfortunately some hospitals are less enthusiastic about allowing female partners and other members of the family in.

Every mother needs to be guided by her inclinations and flexible enough to recognize that her feelings might change during the course of her pregnancy. Family and friends, however much they may want to be there for the big event, should respect your decision to include some and exclude others, as well as your right to amend that decision at any time.

Other Children

For a woman who has other children there is always the nagging question of whether they should attend the birth. There are good arguments for and against this option. Not all childbirth educators believe that having siblings at the birth is a good idea. Children who are young and/or emotionally immature may find it a negative experience, and for some mothers, having a child there can mean she ends up worrying about its welfare rather than letting go and surrendering to the demands of her labour.

However, those who like the idea believe that including other children at the birth contributes greatly to the atmosphere of normalcy and family closeness. If you want your child with you at the birth, issues you should consider are:

• How flexible and prepared you are for labour's demands – your attitude will affect your child's experience.
• Is your practitioner amenable to the idea?
• Does the child want to be there? If not, don't force it. If the child changes its mind at the last minute you must respect this also.
• Can you talk openly about sex and birth to your child and is your child comfortable with a wide range of emotions? Will your child be able to cope if something does go wrong?
• Who will support and take care of your child during labour when you can't?

Remember also to be realistic. Children aren't always overawed by the power and majesty of labour and birth. Be prepared for your child to be childlike, to need someone to wipe a bottom or a nose, to be hungry or grumpy, to say 'no', argue and fuss, to need cuddling and to want to show you something they've just drawn.

Professional Support

Each of the professionals involved in your pregnancy and labour will contribute something, either positively or negatively, to the eventual outcome. If you want a normal or low-tech birth, choose with care.

Obstetrics is the study of abnormal pregnancies, and health service recommendations are that **obstetricians** should limit their involvement to this small minority of women. If your pregnancy is managed by a consultant obstetrician, it will be a medical affair from start to finish.

General practitioners provide the majority of antenatal care in the UK. Care can vary enormously from practice to practice, but in principle GP care is little different from consultant care. The emphasis will be on birth as a medical event. Less than one per cent of GPs will attend a woman in labour – this job is usually left to midwives.

Midwives are specialists in normal pregnancy and birth and there is little doubt that the midwife is the best person to oversee the whole of your pregnancy and birth. They are the only practitioners whose training is based solely on the care and well-being of mothers and their babies.

Under midwifery care mothers are likely to have significantly fewer interventions in labour; most importantly, a lower rate of electronic fetal monitoring, the introduction of which is known to lead to a cascade of other, possibly unnecessary, interventions such as induction and caesarean operations. In addition, mothers are likely to have stronger feelings of empowerment and satisfaction after birth if they have been cared for by a midwife.

Having said this, where a midwife works will affect how she practises. In the hospital setting, midwives can become distracted by the routines of administration such as appointments, assessments and record-keeping. A hospital midwife is expected to carry out the instructions of the obstetrician. For many, their day-to-day job is more like that of a secretary than a health practitioner, and there are those who are never given, and never ask for, more responsibility than this.

Community midwives, who attend home births, may have different motivations. Some still consider midwifery a vocation and are enthusiastic about normal birth. Others are in the community because this is where they have been posted and will bring the hospital with them to whatever setting they work in.

At the other end of the spectrum are midwives who practise privately. **Independent midwives** can provide a total service including antenatal, birth and postnatal care, and are often the best advocates for normal birth. Private midwifery is not cheap – prices range from £2,500 to

£4,000. However, many independent midwives offer schemes which will allow a mother to spread payments over the period of antenatal care and beyond if necessary. You can get a list of the independent midwives in your area by contacting the Independent Midwives Association.

Another kind of 'professional' from the private sector is the **doula**, sometimes called a birth sister. A doula is a trained female birth partner. Ideally she will have had children of her own and will have undergone extensive training in both the physiology and psychology of birthing.

A female companion has long been accepted as the best kind of 'medicine' in labour and doulas are becoming increasingly popular as birth companions. Even today, researchers find that outcomes improve if a doula is present. In one study, the presence of a doula was shown to cut the average length of labour, from admission to delivery, by half (from 19.3 hours to 8.8 hours!).

Don't let the romance of having a doula cloud your mind, however. Doula training can be patchy. To be confident you should look for someone whose training lasted more than a weekend or two and who understands the need for, and has experience of, acting as an advocate for the mother's wishes in a hospital setting.

The organization Birth and Bonding International can provide a list of doulas in your local area.

MAKING LABOUR EASIER

Once the practicalities of arranging a birth are more or less dealt with, you will have a number of other things to consider. Many women are led to believe that labour is an accident waiting to happen. Forget what you've seen in the movies, this rarely happens. What is more, women have a great many more personal resources than they realize and can employ many effective self-help strategies to help ensure that their labour is not overwhelmingly painful, long or risky.

Of these, freedom of movement is one of the most important. Freedom of movement encourages uncomplicated labours and surveys show that when a woman is given the freedom to move around she will use it well and adopt several different positions, particularly during the second stage of labour.

A woman who has the freedom to move around during the early stages of labour and who can take up whatever positions feel best during the second, pushing stage of labour, is doing for herself what the whole range of obstetric drugs claim to do for her. She is helping to strengthen her contractions, to make them more efficient, and to reduce her level of pain.

The table on page 86 shows the pros and cons of conventional forms of labour management. Below are some of the better alternatives.

Staying Upright

In spite of all the evidence against it, lying down, known as the lithotomy position, continues to be the standard policy in many of our maternity units, even though it decreases the flow of blood to the placenta and risks fetal distress. When a woman lies down she is also decreasing the amount of blood available to the uterus – and less blood means less powerful contractions. In addition, because the uterus tilts forward during contractions, a woman who is on her back or even semi-reclining, is making this powerful muscle work twice as hard to achieve the same results.

In women the coccyx, or tailbone, is hinged in order to increase the dimensions of the pelvis during labour. Lying down, leaning back or sitting on your backside means the potential size of the pelvic outlet is reduced by up to 30 per cent.

In contrast, women who choose to give birth in an upright position take fewer pain-relieving drugs and fewer drugs to speed up labour. They also have fewer epidurals and fewer unnecessary caesareans. Women in an upright position also report more satisfaction with the birth process and a greater feeling of having been in control.

Japanese women like to have their leg muscles massaged during labour. They believe that leg muscles are linked to the vagina and pelvic floor. If the leg muscles are relaxed then the vaginal muscles will relax, making birth easier.

The only exception to the never-lie-down rule is lying on your side. Many women find this a comforting and comfortable position to be in, particularly if exhaustion sets in. Available evidence suggests that there is no difference in the length of labour between women in this position and those who remain upright.

Walking in Early Labour

When first-stage contractions become strong enough, many women find that walking, standing or leaning forward are all effective ways of managing the pain. Walking through labour has no known side-effects and is as effective as the artificial hormone syntocinon for strengthening contractions and shortening labour.

This may be because gravity ensures that the weight of the baby is pressing firmly against the cervix. This, in turn, signals the release of the natural hormone oxytocin, improving the regularity and consistency of contractions. Walking also promotes better all-round circulation and, because of this, is ultimately less tiring and painful.

If you're at home, walking around is easy. In hospital it can be harder to organize, especially if you are attached to a drip or monitor. Although walking the corridors or finding an excuse to go to the toilet frequently can be helpful, staff often insist on the mother staying put and using a bedpan. If you are in hospital and you want to stay mobile, you or your partner may have to be very firm.

USING THE BIRTH BALL

The use of the birth ball – a large gymnastic rubber ball – comes from Alexander Technique practitioners. The birth ball has several advantages over other paraphernalia such as bean bags and birth stools. It is more supportive than a bean bag and softer to sit on than a birth stool. The mother can lean over it, sit on it and rotate her hips, even bounce lightly on it. Because it looks like a giant child's ball it evokes a sense of playfulness at a time when the mother may be quite tense.

You can purchase birth balls from a number of sources, including NCT (the National Childbirth Trust). They are usually under £20 and can continue to be useful after birth for relaxation and gentle stretching exercise.

Squatting

The squatting position has become the subject of a lot of jokes involving kaftan-wearing, lentil-eating earth mother types. Go ahead and laugh, but the squatting position is one of the earliest recorded positions for birth and is depicted in paintings of childbearing which date back several millennia before Christ. One of the reasons for all the jokes is that many 'civilized' women find this a really difficult position to get into and maintain. A less active lifestyle, high-heeled shoes and even sitting on toilets instead of squatting, mean that our ankles have largely lost their strength and flexibility.

In older, more traditional societies it is quite common for women to give birth squatting or standing, either supported by their attendants or supporting themselves by means of a rope or bar. By taking up this position a woman can enlarge the pelvic opening by as much as 20 to 30 per cent.

There are only a couple of cautions to consider with the traditional squatting position. Some women find it a difficult and unstable position to take up, and deep squatting can occasionally be very painful and lead to perineal tears. By taking up a supported squat, either holding onto your birth partner(s) or onto a bed or similarly stable piece of furniture, you can avoid both these problems.

Labouring in Water

Many women feel instinctively drawn to water during pregnancy and when in labour. Warm water can be very soothing, and while it will not take the pain of labour away completely, it will soften it and make it more manageable.

There seems to be some indication that, especially for first-time mothers – the group which is on the receiving end of most interventions – labouring in water may actually reduce levels of pain to such a degree that they use significantly fewer drugs. For instance, in one survey of a group of first-time mothers labouring in water, only 24 per cent used pain-relieving drugs compared to 50 per cent of those labouring out of water.

The safety of labour and birth in water is well-demonstrated and may not have so much to do with what the water does as what the water

Eating for Labour

During labour you will be doing the hardest, most physical job of your life. Denied proper fuel, your muscles cannot work efficiently. The uterus is a muscle and glucose provides the energy which it and all your other muscles need while working so hard. If the body is short of glucose because of fasting it will burn other fuel, such as fat. If this goes on for some time you become ketotic. Ketones – the acidic products of fat metabolism – accumulate in the blood and are a sign of profound exhaustion. They are toxic and can put you and your baby at risk.

Nevertheless, most hospitals refuse women food and drink in labour, preferring instead to keep them artificially hydrated and their blood sugar levels up by using an intravenous drip of water and glucose (also known as dextrose).

The accepted reason for this is 'just in case' a general anaesthetic is needed. Under these circumstances, medics argue, there is a risk a mother might inhale her own vomit, resulting in respiratory problems and occasionally death. More and more this policy is being questioned. Studies show that the stomach is never truly empty anyway, and that for pregnant women the benefits of eating and drinking as they wish may outweigh any theoretical risk. Also, it is not the food but the skill of the anaesthetist which causes problems. If a woman has been properly anaesthetized, there is no reason why she should inhale her own vomit. In any case, the general anaesthetic is used so rarely today that it hardly justifies the widespread policy of starvation during labour.

Although many women do not want to eat, particularly in the later stages of labour, the choice of eating and drinking freely, especially early on, should be entirely theirs. If you are at home the choice is already yours. If you are planning to give birth in hospital and feel strongly about this issue, you may have to insist on bringing your own food from home. Suitable choices include:
• fruit juices
• bananas
• herbal tea with honey
• clear broth (e.g. miso)

- crispbreads, breadsticks or rice cakes
- toast, lightly buttered or with honey
- lightly boiled or scrambled eggs
- cooked fruits such as apple sauce
- glucose tablets (for when you really need quick energy)

represents. Basically, a mother who is labouring or birthing in water is much harder to interfere with. Enclosed within the boundaries of the pool she is more protected and autonomous; she can't easily be fitted with tubes and belts or jabbed with needles. The low rates of intervention for women who labour and give birth in water are testimony to this. It may also be that doctors and midwives, in the presence of a woman who feels secure and who is labouring in a self-possessed manner, feel less inclined to interfere.

NEARLY THERE

It seems unfair that the business of giving birth isn't over until the placenta is safely delivered. This is a stage of labour which many women never think about. In their minds the placenta is just the bloody 'afterbirth', not the miraculous organ which kept their baby alive for all those months.

But even at this final stage, unnecessary medical intervention can complicate rather than assist labour. The usual routine is to give the mother an injection of syntometrine as soon as the baby is delivered and to use a

Your placenta is your property – why not take a look at it? For many women the shape and structure of the placenta reminds them of a tree. For nine long months its various branches have delivered food and removed waste from your baby's body. By the end of your pregnancy the branching vessels of this very special tree of life will have become so numerous that their total surface would cover more than half a tennis court. If you wish to make a ritual with your placenta such as burying it under a specially planted tree in the garden, you can ask the midwife to put it aside for you to take away with you when you leave hospital.

combination of pulling on the umbilical cord and pressing hard on the mother's abdomen to speed the separation of the placenta from the uterine wall.

Mounting evidence, however, suggests that medical management of the third stage of labour doesn't prevent the problems it is supposed to. Syntometrine does not prevent post-partum haemorrhage (though it is effective in stopping it once it has occurred) and used in conjunction with pulling on the cord it is, in reality, a major cause of this problem. What is more, because the cord will need to be clamped early, usually before it has stopped pulsing, in order to prevent the drug from reaching your baby, the baby will be denied its full complement of blood. When the cord is cut too early there may not be enough blood in your baby's body to support the circulatory system. Under these circumstances the body will divert blood from elsewhere such as the respiratory system, leaving the lungs under-inflated.

The kinder (to mother and baby) alternative is to allow the third stage to unfold in the same unhurried way as the birth of your baby. In a normal, physiological third stage the placenta is delivered by the mother, with the aid of gravity and in its own time. It is perfectly normal for as much as an hour to pass after the baby is born before the placenta makes its appearance. Putting your baby to the breast and altering your position to a more upright one will help ensure the safe completion of the third stage.

CHAPTER 7

SPECIAL CONDITIONS

For some women, being pregnant can give rise to certain health conditions which are unique to pregnancy. For others it may aggravate or complicate pre-existing health problems. This does not always mean, however, that the woman cannot have a normal pregnancy and delivery if this is what she desires. Even if you do have a pre-existing health condition, don't be too quick to assign yourself to a high-risk category. Even the insulin-dependent diabetic can have a more or less normal pregnancy provided she is motivated and given good support and accurate information about how to keep her diabetes under control. Equally, although women with multiple sclerosis are often told they are high risk, this diagnosis seems to defy the laws of biology. MS is a disease of the central nervous system. Unless our bodies have changed drastically in the last few decades, the uterus is not affected at all by dysfunction in this area (even paraplegic women have normally functioning reproductive organs!).

What many doctors forget is that for a woman with an existing health complaint it may be even more important to her, emotionally and psychologically, to keep medical intervention to a minimum. In such a woman, faith in her body may already be at an all-time low. A birth experience which the woman feels she has had some contribution to can go a long way towards restoring that faith. All too many of the drugs and procedures used in modern antenatal and labour management can make health problems worse. For instance, the pain-relieving drugs can trigger an attack in asthmatic women. The glucose and insulin drip used to control the blood sugar of a diabetic woman in labour can all too easily disrupt, rather than maintain, her blood sugar level.

If for any reason you do need to rely upon medical management to see you through pregnancy and birth, this is not a failure on your part. There is still a great deal you can do to complement medical care, such as paying close attention to your diet, taking regular exercise and following the suggestions in the preceding chapter to reduce the toxic load on your body. You may wish to discuss your options for alternative care with more than one practitioner, including your GP, your midwife and your chosen alternative practitioner(s). Many alternative therapies can be used to lessen the severity of conditions such as herpes and Strep-b infection. An holistic approach now may help maintain a better biochemical balance in your body and for some it may provide a way to lower dependence on certain drugs which may pose a threat to your developing child. In fact, exploring a wide range of options may be even more important to the women who needs some degree of medical care, since these may help restore some of her sense of control over her own life and that of her child.

Problems of Metabolism

Some of the most common pregnancy-related problems can be attributed to faulty metabolism. Briefly defined, metabolism is how your body takes in food and converts it into essential energy and nutrients which feed you and your baby.

The organ most involved in metabolism, and the one which probably comes under the most stress during pregnancy, is your liver. The liver is the largest internal organ in the body and is responsible for enriching the blood with nutrients, removing toxins and converting and storing energy from your food. As pregnancy progresses and the baby's demands for energy and nutrients become greater, it is important that you do all you can to support this important organ.

In grouping together the three main problems of metabolism: anaemia, gestational diabetes and pre-eclampsia, we begin to see that these are not simply isolated diseases which strike the pregnant woman for no apparent reason, but messages from her body telling her that it is getting too much or not enough of something.

Anaemia

The symptoms of anaemia – tiredness, shortness of breath, dizzy spells and becoming easily exhausted after strenuous activity – are difficult to distinguish from the common symptoms of pregnancy. The only way to tell for sure if you are anaemic is to have a blood test, and even then the results are open to wide interpretation. The normal range of haemoglobin in the blood is 13–15 grams per decilitre at less than 8 weeks' gestation. This drops naturally to between 10–12 g/dl from about 28 weeks' gestation.

The reason your practitioner may be concerned is that there are risks in pregnancy and labour associated with profound anaemia. The woman's contractions may be more painful and less efficient, she may be more prone to heavy bleeding, and she is more vulnerable to post-partum infection. For the baby it means that there is less oxygen in the blood, which can result in poor growth and premature labour. In spite of this, it is very unlikely that a woman who is told her iron levels are low is actually anaemic.

During pregnancy the baby's needs take priority, so iron and other nutrients are first diverted to the placenta. This is offset, in part, by the fact that the woman is not losing blood from her monthly periods. It is only if the mother's levels of iron are initially very low that she will begin to suffer.

The body chemistry of a healthy woman changes throughout pregnancy to allow greater absorption of iron. At 36 weeks her body's ability to absorb iron is nine times greater than in early pregnancy. This means that, given a good diet, the body is quite capable of keeping both mother and baby healthy during pregnancy. It may even be that a drop in iron levels is a normal adaptation of pregnancy. Certainly there is evidence that women with low iron levels during pregnancy tend to have bigger, healthier babies.

The chemistry of your body is very delicately balanced, so, before trying to boost your iron levels artificially with supplements, consider the potential problems they can cause. Synthetic irons can cause constipation, nausea, dizziness and diarrhoea and are less easily absorbed, placing greater strain on your body. Vomiting and diarrhoea can further deplete the body's stores of iron. Iron gained from a nutritious diet produces no such side-effects. If your iron levels are on the low side of normal, consider the dietary measures outlined in chapter 3 first. Consider also having a glass of citrus juice with each meal to aid absorption of iron from your food.

Gestational Diabetes

Gestational diabetes is often used to explain the fact that a woman has produced a large baby. Such a woman may be told that her baby is more likely to get stuck during birth (known as shoulder dystocia) and that she should have a caesarean to avert such a likelihood. There is no evidence that this is a reasonable course of action. Some babies are simply big and as pregnancy progresses ultrasound becomes an increasingly inaccurate tool for predicting birthweight. The size of your baby has nothing to do with it getting 'stuck' – more than half of the babies who do get stuck are of a 'normal' size.

Many practitioners are now beginning to believe that the search for gestational diabetes – dubbed by some as a collection of symptoms looking for a disease – is a pointless exercise.

Because so many women are afraid of producing 'big' babies, or rather are afraid of how they are going to get a 'big' baby out, the diagnosis of gestational diabetes can be particularly anxiety-provoking. Some women just make large babies, and other possible influences such as the birthweight of both parents, the woman's pre-pregnant weight, her weight gain during pregnancy, the quality of her diet and whether or not the pregnancy might be post-term are likely to be more influential than any change in her blood glucose levels.

Even though there is no clear definition of gestational diabetes, once diagnosed it places a woman in a 'high-risk' category, which will mean greater anxiety for her and more 'routine' tests. It is hard to say with any certainty what 'normal' blood sugar levels are in pregnancy, though they are certainly different (probably higher) than in non-pregnant women. Your best course of action is to focus on the solution instead of the 'problem'.

The best way to maintain a level uptake of glucose is to eat a well-balanced wholefood diet. If your blood glucose levels are still on the high side of normal, consider taking extra exercise and being extra careful about hidden sugars such as those in 'healthy' fruit juices. Cutting out fruit juice altogether and opting for water and herb teas may make a big difference.

Pre-eclampsia

This condition affects between 5 and 10 per cent of women to varying degrees. A diagnosis of pre-eclampsia *must* be based on the presence of hypertension (raised blood pressure), oedema (swelling due to water retention) and raised levels of uric acid in the blood. When these symptoms are present together they usually indicate pre-eclampsia. On their own, any one of them is unlikely to indicate a substantial problem.

Pre-eclampsia is more common in first pregnancies and usually shows itself in middle to late pregnancy (except in women who have been malnourished for years). Women who have diabetes or kidney disease, high blood pressure, twins or more, those with a family history of high blood pressure or a previous pre-eclamptic pregnancy, women over 40, those who suffer from migraine and those who had pre-eclampsia in a previous pregnancy, are most at risk.

A woman's partner also seems to have some influence. Provided she is with the same partner, her chance of developing pre-eclampsia declines with each pregnancy. However, if a woman has her second or subsequent baby with a different man, the chances of developing pre-eclampsia are the same as if she were having her first baby. The risk is even higher if she is with man who has already fathered a child whose mother suffered from pre-eclampsia.

But perhaps the single most consistent factor linked to pre-eclampsia is poor diet, giving rise to the idea that pre-eclampsia has a metabolic origin. A number of studies show that it is more likely to develop in women who are very undernourished and living in a stressful environment.

Some doctors still consider this point of view to be controversial. Nevertheless, there is a large body of evidence to suggest that only those practitioners who have paid close attention to the diets of the women in their care have achieved substantial reductions, and in some cases completely eliminated, pre-eclampsia from their practices.

Certainly, while doctors also use a number of drugs to combat pre-eclampsia and keep it from developing into full-blown eclampsia, there is much less convincing evidence that any of these actually do much good. In response to this midwives, and some self-help organizations, usually recommend women try following what is known as the Brewer Diet devised by the American obstetrician, Dr Tom Brewer.

Rereading Brewer's original material is enlightening, since his recommendations, made 25 years ago, are very much in line with the current healthy eating guidelines in both the US and UK. The only exception is that Dr Brewer recommended that pregnant women needed an extra serving of meat or similar complete protein and an extra serving of dairy products each day. Provided she is not suffering from any other disorder which affects her liver function, a pregnant woman should consider taking in an increased amount of protein (animal or vegetable) along with a diet high in wholefoods (and low in refined foods) to ensure that her body systems are functioning optimally. The group PETS (the Pre-eclampsia Society) can provide more information on the Brewer Diet.

Although your doctor or midwife may be able to diagnose pre-eclampsia, they are unlikely to be able to suggest a cure apart from an early caesarean and drugs to control the symptoms. Also while doctors sometimes use dietary manipulations with regard to pre-eclampsia, these usually involve restrictions. For instance, during your antenatal care you may be advised to limit both your salt and fluid intake in order to prevent pre-eclampsia. This is advice has *no scientific backing*. Pregnant women should salt to their taste and drink to their thirst. Restricting your fluid intake, in particular, will not prevent the water retention associated with pre-eclampsia. Between 50 and 80 per cent of pregnant women experience some form of water retention and swelling, usually in the ankles, feet, hands and face. Free intake of fluids keeps your kidneys working well, and flushes waste products out of your system – again benefiting you and your baby.

All this does not mean that you should ignore the signs of genuine pre-eclampsia. Left untreated, pre-eclampsia poses a threat to your baby. The placenta will not be functioning at its optimum level and the baby is at risk of poor growth. Unable to support the baby's growth your body may well initiate premature labour.

Further, for a rare few women, pre-eclampsia can develop into full-blown eclampsia – a potentially lethal condition for mother and baby. Early symptoms include severe headaches, flashing lights, nausea, vomiting and pain in the abdomen. In very extreme cases the mother may experience fits, convulsions and, more rarely, go into a coma. If you are experiencing any of these symptoms get yourself to the hospital immediately for testing.

In mild to moderate form, though, pre-eclampsia may not affect the course of your labour. However, it's probably even more important that you feel relaxed and happy about the environment in which you are giving birth, since stress can aggravate the symptoms of pre-eclampsia. You may be advised to have an epidural during labour because of the way it lowers blood pressure. For some this is reasonable advice which allows them to labour and give birth without resorting to surgery.

Placenta Praevia

When the placenta is covering the opening of the cervix this is known as placenta praevia. A caesarean will be necessary since your baby will not be able to be born vaginally. That's the not-so-good news.

The better news is that early pronouncements of a 'low-lying placenta' detected by ultrasound are generally unreliable. In early pregnancy many women have placentas which appear to be lying low enough to indicate the risk of placenta praevia. The vast majority of these move out of the way as the uterus grows larger. Don't be tempted to have a scan every few weeks to see if you still have a low-lying placenta. Wait until later in pregnancy and then check again if you are at all worried.

If your placenta is still in the way your biggest decision is when you will have the caesarean. Most doctors would recommend that you have it well before term, between 36 and 38 weeks, but this may be unnecessarily aggressive. The longer your baby can remain inside you the better. There is evidence to show that in women whose placenta praevia was not diagnosed until labour, the outcomes were just as good as those who had theirs diagnosed early. That is to say their babies were delivered safely by caesarean and none of the women or babies died as a result of going into labour with this condition.

Each case must be judged on its own merits. With placenta praevia you may experience some bleeding as you get closer to term. This is caused by the tearing of the placenta as the cervix stretches. The bleeding is unlikely to be heavy. Instead it may come in small brown clumps and often

TESTING THE WATERS

Your baby is swimming around in a warm liquid called the amniotic fluid. How much fluid can vary enormously between individual women and there is also a wide range of medically defined 'norms'. Nevertheless, today many practitioners routinely check for amniotic fluid volume when they scan a mother. As a result, far too many women today are being told they have 'too little' or 'too much' amniotic fluid.

Amniotic fluid volume tends to increase during the early part of pregnancy and remains stable from about 26 to 38 weeks. Towards the end of pregnancy, levels gradually begin to decrease. During labour, very low levels may increase the risk of pressure on the umbilical cord during contractions and this in turn can cause fetal distress due to lack of oxygen. Ironically, breaking a woman's waters in early labour creates the same risk, though this fact rarely stops midwives from doing it!

Remember that 'too little' and 'too much' can be opinions rather than diagnoses. A second opinion from another practitioner might yield an entirely different result. In addition, once they have offered this opinion, doctors rarely have any help to offer you except induction, performing an early caesarean or asking you to come in for weekly (or more frequent) scans. Indeed, too little fluid is increasingly used as a way of leading the mother towards an induction.

Consider this: fetal swallowing and urinating account for about 50 per cent of your amniotic fluid. The rest is up to you. Maternal hydration has a significant role to play in keeping up your levels of amniotic fluid. One study showed that when women who had oligohydramnios (too little amniotic fluid) drank two litres of water prior to having a scan their amniotic fluid volume rose by between 8 and 16 per cent – enough to avert any potential problems. So if you are told that your amniotic fluid volume is low, consider whether your fluid intake is adequate.

The risks of too much amniotic fluid (polyhydramnios) are less clear. High levels of fluid are sometimes associated with fetal abnormalities and may increase the risk of post-partum haemorrhage due to over-extension of the uterus.

These problems are somewhat theoretical and there is little you can do about this condition anyway. Instead, focus on your total health and make sure that you pay attention to those things which might interfere with your body's total water balance. This means avoiding caffeinated drinks and sodas and opting instead for plenty of water, grain coffees and herbal teas.

it stops for long periods of time. As long as the baby shows no signs of compromise you could consider a watch-and-wait approach until you are as near term as you feel comfortable with. The choice should be yours.

CAN I STILL HAVE A NORMAL BIRTH?

Occasionally, health problems which were present before a woman became pregnant can make having a totally normal birth difficult. The extent to which they will become a determining factor in the course of your pregnancy and labour really depends on the extent of the condition itself. Many disorders such as asthma and hypertension can be made worse by the hormonal and emotional changes of pregnancy and will need to be carefully monitored by the mother and her practitioner. This does not mean, however, that you will need more medical care. Learn the difference between monitoring – which is essentially non-active – and care, which denotes active management. There is insufficient space in this book to cover all the alternative ways of working with the conditions listed below. A great deal of literature exists in libraries and bookshops and through specialist organizations. The mother suffering from any of the following is advised to seek this out in order to minimize the impact of her pregnancy on her health and vice versa.

Asthma

This condition can sometimes be made worse by pregnancy. This may be because the root cause of the asthma is some allergen in your immediate environment, either at home or work. Food allergy is also a possibility. During pregnancy your body will be having to deal with an increased amount of waste products and for some there is the possibility of overload. Asthma is also made worse by anxiety so attacks may mirror moments of fear and doubt.

A good first step would be to consider having yourself tested for sensitivity to food and environmental allergens. Groups such as Foresight and the British Society of Allergy, Environmental and Nutritional Medicine can help with this. It is also particularly useful if you can engage in exercises which emphasize breathing out, such as yoga. Not only will such regular activity relax you, but it can help retrain your breathing. Many non-drug methods of dealing with asthma, such as the Buteko method, emphasize the importance of a full outbreath. By fully emptying your lungs you are exercising all the tiny bronchi and helping to maintain their elasticity. You are also blowing out toxins which collect in your lungs.

It is particularly important for asthmatics to try to avoid narcotics during labour. The pain relievers commonly used in hospitals will depress your breathing further, placing your baby at greater risk. Consider trying other ways of managing, such as using water for labour and/or birth and remaining mobile and changing positions frequently during labour.

Diabetes

If you are an insulin-dependent diabetic you will probably need to re-educate yourself about diabetes and its control, especially during the first few months of pregnancy. At first it may be difficult to control your diabetes but you will soon learn that control is achievable through multiple measures such as diet and exercise as well as your insulin injections. Things usually settle down in the second trimester and beyond.

Your physician's main concern will be the effect which pregnancy has on your kidneys, heart and eyes as well as the link between diabetes and very large babies. Diabetes is also associated with a higher than normal risk of fetal abnormalities and miscarriage. As explained earlier, a huge baby is not a given in a diabetic pregnancy, so don't be panicked into lots of scans to continually check the size of your baby. Scans to determine the size of the baby are not usually very accurate after about 18 weeks so there is little point in going through the motions. You may be relieved to know that the risk of passing on your diabetes to your child is very small, less than 2 per cent.

Your doctor will probably advise you to have an elective caesarean before term. This is likely to be an unnecessarily aggressive solution. The majority of studies into this subject have shown that bringing the pregnancy to an artificial end, either through caesarean or induction, is unlikely to be of demonstrable benefit for the mother or her baby. If you are otherwise healthy and your pregnancy has been uncomplicated, you can and should expect to give birth to your baby yourself.

Whether it will be a 'normal' delivery is another thing. Debate rages about whether diabetic women should have the full range of interventions including a glucose drip, to help them in labour. It is unreasonable to assume that a glucose drip will control a mother's blood sugar any better than eating and drinking freely and regularly monitoring her blood sugar. Some diabetic women under the care of skilled midwives have coped perfectly well in this way. Nevertheless, great pressure will be brought to bear on you to have the drip instead of the food. The choice should be entirely yours, but usually it is not unless you opt for a home or similarly low-tech birth.

Remember that how your body uses glucose will depend on many things. Your level of anxiety will affect insulin levels. Giving birth in a reclining position will make your muscles work harder and therefore also cause a dramatic change in blood sugar levels. If you are diabetic you should arrange beforehand to be upright and supported throughout your labour. Using a water pool to control the pain will also help.

Genital Herpes

The risks of this viral infection vary according to the mother's own history of the disease. If this is your first herpes infection of any kind (known as primary genital herpes) your baby is at greater risk simply because you lack the antibodies necessary to fight the infection. Primary genital herpes is associated with greater risk of miscarriage, and illness in the baby, including skin lesions and congenital malformations. There is a higher rate of premature birth and low birthweight infants when primary infection occurs after 20 weeks' gestation.

A baby born to a mother with primary lesions (open sores which shed the virus) is at greater risk of developing meningitis and possibly dying.

A blood test is crucial to determine if your condition is primary or not.

Non-primary genital herpes indicates a woman who has previously had herpes at another site in her body but who has developed genital symptoms for the first time. Recurrent genital herpes denotes a woman who has a prior history of genital outbreaks. The baby is less at risk because the mother will have already developed antibodies to the virus. This immunity can be passed onto the baby, lessening the impact of the disease on the child at birth. It is impossible to predict which babies might contract the disease and which will not.

Antibiotics will not help because herpes is a virus. Effective alternative methods include taking zinc with each meal. Start at a low dose of 25mg and work your way up to a maximum of around 250mg three times a day (it is important to find the right level for you since there are individual levels above which zinc can cause nausea in some people). Foods with arginine (an amino acid which feeds the herpes virus) such as nuts, nut products, pork, chocolate and coffee should be avoided. Opt instead for food rich in lysine, such as dairy products, poultry, fish and eggs. Seek the help of a qualified homeopath or herbalist and make sure you balance adequate amounts of exercise and rest. You should also increase your intake of B-vitamins.

Heart Problems

Your heart comes under more strain during pregnancy. It will grow bigger and be pumping a greater volume of blood around your body. The extra weight you are carrying may also be a factor. If you suffer from a heart condition such as arrhythmia or hypertension you should do all that you can to protect and assist your heart during this time.

Your physician's concern is that your baby should continue to get enough oxygen, via the blood to the placenta, and that the extra strain on your heart should not cause your condition to deteriorate. The kind of pregnancy and birth you have will depend on the extent to which your heart or circulatory health has already deteriorated. If you suffer from mild to moderate heart or circulatory problems and have managed to bring this under control with dietary and lifestyle modifications, there is no reason why you should not continue confidently along this path while pregnant. If you are taking drugs to control any number of heart symptoms you may wish to discuss the choice of medications with your physician early on. Some drugs are less safe for your baby than others. For instance, beta-blockers can be used to control hypertension in the third trimester of pregnancy, but used early on are associated with a risk of growth retardation.

How to maintain your health at this time will depend on your health pre-pregnancy. If you have been fairly active and incorporated an exercise regime into your life before conception then you should continue to do so now. If not, now is not the time to begin vigorous exercise. Instead, opt for gentle regimes such as swimming and yoga, which will both calm and invigorate the body. If you are a person who is tense, stress management techniques may be useful now. Anger and anxiety can have a profound effect on blood pressure and heart health. So can loneliness and feeling disconnected from others – so seek support whenever and wherever you can.

Your diet will be very important. Make sure your intake of vitamins C and E are adequate and that you stick to what is known as the Mediterranean diet – one which is high in fresh fruits and vegetables which act as protective anti-oxidants. The Mediterranean diet is also high in 'good' fats such as sunflower oil – a rich source of protective omega-3 fatty acids, and olive oil – a mono-saturated oil which is particularly suitable for cooking since it can withstand high temperatures without producing toxic byproducts known as free radicals.

Multiple Sclerosis

For some women this condition can be aggravated by pregnancy. But others report feeling much better, especially after the first few months when morning sickness is not so much of a problem.

Some of the symptoms which you experience during pregnancy may simply be that – symptoms of pregnancy, so don't worry that your condition is deteriorating if, for example, you are running to the toilet more often than usual.

Although you will be put in a 'high-risk' category, MS generally causes few problems in pregnancy or labour. In fact, research into MS and pregnancy recently came to the unexpected conclusion that pregnancy may actually delay relapses in the condition. The suggestion is that circulating levels of alpha-fetoprotein may have a suppressive effect.

If you were taking nutritional supplements such as vitamins, minerals and evening primrose oil before pregnancy, you should continue to take these now. There is no need to increase your dose. If you have not been taking B-complex up until now, it might be a good idea to include this as a daily supplement during pregnancy. Make sure your supplement includes between 25 and 50ug/mcg of B12.

MS is a disease of the central nervous system; it does not affect your uterus in any way. The biggest problem you will have to face in labour is that labour is tiring. However, unless you are very incapacitated to begin with, you should be free to choose whatever type of birth you would like. It may be difficult, however, to persuade your doctor or midwife of the fact that high-tech management is inappropriate.

Choosing an atmosphere which is stress-free will help prevent extreme fatigue. If you find the idea of water in labour relaxing, go for a water birth. Make sure you can eat and drink freely to keep your energy levels up during labour. In fact, should you wish to give birth at home or at a birth centre, this may be your best choice. Women with MS who have had normal births report feelings of great satisfaction with themselves and their bodies (something which should not be underestimated with a disease which makes you feel like your body is at war with you). If this is what you want, however, be prepared to put up a struggle.

Strep-b

Strep-b is a chronic infection caused by the streptococcus bacteria. Because of the overuse of antibiotics in our society, not just as human medicines but in the foods we eat as well, there is often no way to cure it completely once a person is infected.

Any chronic infection suggests a poorly functioning immune system. Many things can adversely affect your immune system, including over-use of medications and a diet which includes foods which you are allergic to or which are high in toxins such as pesticides. Mothers with Strep-b may be at increased risk of miscarriage and pre-term birth. It can also lead to inflammation of the amniotic sac, the uterine lining or the urinary tract of the mother.

The infection can be passed onto the baby at birth but antibiotic treatment during pregnancy will not necessarily prevent this from occurring. So, if you are asymptomatic, you may wish to consider other options such as supplemental echinacea root tincture, which has been shown in several scientific studies to be effective against both Staph and Strep bacteria.

You will be advised to have a medically directed birth which may include either induction before term or a caesarean. Consider these options carefully. Induction will place an enormous strain on your body and caesarean raises your risk of developing a post-surgical infection. Your body simply may not be able to cope. The most common protocol in hospitals is to give the mother large doses of antibiotics during labour in the hope that these will reach her baby and prevent the bacteria from taking hold. Again, this is by no means 100 per cent foolproof.

Spontaneous rupture of the membranes does not appear to increase the risk for the baby provided birth occurs within 18 hours, especially if the infant is at full term and is the product of a well-nourished mother. Boosting your vitamin C intake to at least 500mg daily will help strengthen the amniotic sac and thus prevent early rupture of the membranes.

Taking care of yourself is not an option here. You should consider having yourself tested for food allergies and vitamin deficiencies – preferably before conception. Switching to organic, or the best-quality food you can afford, should also be a priority. A qualified herbalist or homeopath may be able to suggest ways of supporting and strengthening your immune system during pregnancy and beyond.

Strep-b is often found in women who have candida problems. An intestine infested with candida may be more vulnerable to colonization by this aggressive bacterium. A totally sugar-free diet will help enormously (and this includes no fruit juices or other 'natural' sugars).

Since infection and reinfection are possible through sexual contact, consider using a condom.

PART II
THE THERAPIES

CHAPTER 8

CHOOSING A THERAPY

Natural is best – right? The answer is a qualified 'yes'. Qualified, not because there is anything inherently dangerous about alternative medicine, but because every time you put something in your mouth, every time you manipulate the spine, massage a muscle or stimulate an acupoint, you are producing change in your body. Most of the time these changes will be beneficial.

Alternative remedies can claim success in treating a wide range of conditions. Acupuncture, aromatherapy, herbalism, homeopathy and various forms of massage have all been shown, through research and anecdote, to be beneficial in pregnancy and birth. Most can be chosen with confidence to deal with minor physical aches and pains and some can be effective in easing emotional anxieties.

What is more, while some therapies such as osteopathy, acupuncture, chiropractic and more advanced herbal medicine require the participation of a highly trained and experienced therapist, others, such as homeopathy, self-massage, simple aromatherapy and nutritional measures, can be simply and safely applied as a form of 'self-help'. Alternative therapies, therefore, offer two important services to pregnant women: they are generally safe and effective and some offer ways of self-treatment which can increase a woman's confidence in her ability to care effectively for herself and her baby.

However, while natural alternatives are unlikely to cause great harm, in unskilled hands they are capable of causing ill-effects. Many natural remedies can be extremely powerful and, no matter what any therapist tells you, no remedy or treatment can be both powerful and totally benign. Anything capable of producing profound positive change can also produce profound negative change in some individuals.

Occasionally, for example, you may experience a temporary trade-off of symptoms, or side-effects which are unexpected and unpleasant. Some therapists refer to this as a 'healing crisis'. Often, you will be told that sickness, pain and fatigue are a good sign – a sign that the body is healing itself. While there may be some truth in this, it is also reminiscent of the purging and puking ideas of Victorian medicine. A prolonged healing crisis is not really appropriate at any time but especially not during pregnancy, when it can be debilitating and risk the health of both the mother and her child.

The conventional approach to healing encourages the 'patient' to switch off and leave everything to the experts. Often we take this attitude with us when we make the shift to an alternative therapy. A more positive way of approaching alternatives, however, is to consider that they provide a unique opportunity to break out of this negative pattern and take charge of your own health.

Consider also that it is not just women who 'switch off' when they enter the world of alternative medicine. Some alternative practitioners also bring conventional ideas with them into their practices. Alternative therapists and holistic midwives can be unbelievably quick to interfere with, or try to alter, the natural course of pregnancy and birth. Some may opt to start their clients on 'natural' labour preparations, usually herbal tinctures or homeopathic remedies, from around 34 to 36 weeks. Often there is no reason to suspect that the woman is at risk from a problem labour or being 'overdue' and there is absolutely no indication that such interventions are of genuine value.

The justification for such actions is usually something like, 'I have been doing this for several years and I've never had a woman go significantly past her due date.' This is a fallacious justification for interference. Without the aid of herbs, potions and powders the same practitioner may find that women under his or her care still do not go significantly past their due dates.

The therapies and medicines covered in the chapters which follow have all been shown to be effective in one way or another during pregnancy and for the labouring woman. However, they should be used sensitively and intelligently and not as a crutch – for either mother or practitioner – or a talisman to help create the illusion of control over a process which is largely out of our control.

Although alternative medicine breaks many of convention's rules, one golden rule still applies: 'First do no harm'. This rule relates to more than just the physical body; it applies to the psyche as well. If a remedy becomes just another emotional or psychological crutch, then a therapist has done just as much damage to the woman in his or her care as if they had given her a synthetic drug.

Many of the medicines, alternative or otherwise, which we use to treat pregnancy complaints are simply making up for poor diet and a stressful life. If every condition is met with a magic bullet approach, rather than information, support and suggestions for lifestyle changes, we are simply encouraging women to substitute one system of pill popping for another.

Happily, the majority of alternative practitioners do encourage their clients to become partners in their own health. Once you have done this, you will never view the conventional system of care in the same way. Having accepted responsibility for their own health, many women find a new confidence to dictate to their conventional practitioners the kind of care they wish to receive during pregnancy, rather than simply being passive recipients of routine care.

If you are new to the use of alternative therapies (and even if you are not) there are some sensible guidelines to consider which may help you to make sense of whether a particular therapy (or a therapist) is the right choice for you.

'What's in it?'

The choice of a therapy or remedy is often highly individual, so don't simply rely on claims and recommendations. Try to make an informed decision and refuse to be passive about the 'stuff' which you are being offered. Detailed information on all the alternative therapies is beyond the scope of this book. However, there exists a wealth of information in libraries and bookshops about all forms of alternative therapies.

Always ask what's in a particular remedy, tincture or pill. Check which oils your aromatherapist is using. These are not trade secrets and should not be treated as such. Ask also what each of the ingredients does and what you can expect from a particular remedy. Any therapist who is reluctant to answer such basic questions should be regarded with suspicion.

It shouldn't hurt

This sounds obvious but it is amazing what some people will put up with! Massage, chiropractic or osteopathy should *never* hurt. If it does, inform your practitioner. If he or she does not listen, get a new practitioner.

Homeopathy, herbs and even massage can sometimes produce unexpected side-effects. These should not be severe and should not last a long time. Some therapists are very enthusiastic about these reactions and encourage their patients to put up with all manner of adverse effects. Pregnancy is not a time to be going through a major 'healing crisis'. If you are unhappy with the effect of a particular therapy and your practitioner does not acknowledge and act upon your feelings, change practitioners. This advice, by the way, also applies to midwives, GPs and obstetricians. You always have the right to switch to someone new if you are unhappy with your care.

Give it time

Alternative therapies do not work in the same way as conventional therapies. Whatever form of therapy you choose, and provided you do not actually feel worse, give it time.

Conventional medicine works, in the main, by suppressing symptoms. Alternative therapies work by addressing the cause and healing the whole body. This process can take time. Bouncing from one practitioner or therapy to another because things aren't moving fast enough is likely to be counter-productive.

Less is more

Generally speaking, you should only take a remedy up to the point where you begin to feel better. The aim of alternative medicine is to support the body's own ability to heal and change, not to undermine it or do all the work for it. Studies into some herbs, for instance, have shown that taking larger amounts does not always produce better or faster results than taking small, regular doses. The same is true for homeopathy, and a good osteopath or reflexologist will know when 'hands off' is better than 'hands on'.

Work with your body

Have some faith that your body can do what it is supposed to. It can make a healthy baby. It can cope with all these tremendous physical changes. It can tell you what is wrong both physically and emotionally if you learn to listen to it. Before you go running to any practitioner, conventional or alternative, spend a few days trying to 'tune in' to your real needs.

Get plenty of rest, eat good food, accept help from others and pay attention to any feelings and intuitions you have. Ask yourself whether your body is talking to you in metaphor. Is your backache telling you to stop 'carrying' so much? Are your chronic headaches a sign to 'get out of your head' and pay closer attention to the demands of your changing body? Are you nauseous because you just can't 'stomach' something any more? If things improve after a few days then you have found a solution, or a beginning of one. If you still feel that you would like extra help then choose a therapy which you feel comfortable with.

Following these simple guidelines should ensure that you get the best out of whatever therapy you choose.

CHAPTER 9

ACUPUNCTURE

--- **WHAT IT'S BEST FOR** ---

NAUSEA

PAIN RELIEF

VARICOSE VEINS

HEARTBURN

HEADACHES/MIGRAINES

CONSTIPATION

DIARRHOEA

HAEMORRHOIDS

DIGESTIVE DISTURBANCES

OEDEMA

TURNING A BREECH

INDUCING LABOUR

LESSENING LABOUR PAINS

ASTHMA

ALLERGIES AND RESPIRATORY PROBLEMS

INSOMNIA

☑ **Requires a professional therapist**

All human life is made of energy ...

This, at least, is one thing upon which holistic practitioners and medical scientists can agree. According to the Chinese, the life energy which surrounds us and flows through us is called Qi or Chi (pronounced *chee*). When this life force is disturbed, either because it is blocked or because it is moving too slowly or too fast, imbalance and eventually illness will result. Acupuncture is a system of healing which aims to restore health by bringing your life energy into balance.

The word acupuncture has two roots in Latin: *acus* meaning needle and *punctura*, to puncture. Like many great discoveries, acupuncture evolved through a mixture of serendipity and science. In China, thousands of years ago, a strange wartime phenomenon was observed; soldiers whose bodies were pierced by arrows sometimes recovered from illnesses which had plagued them for years. Eventually the idea evolved that, by penetrating the skin at certain points, diseases could be cured.

Although acupuncture has been an important part of traditional Chinese medicine for more than 2,500 years, it is only over the last 20 years or so that it has come to be more widely accepted by healthcare practitioners and the general public in the West. Indeed, the World Health Organization (WHO) has gone so far as to state that there is now sufficient medical evidence to support the effectiveness of acupuncture for it to be considered an important part of primary health care. The WHO has also, remarkably, recommended that acupuncture should be fully integrated into conventional medicine.

There are more than 2,000 acupuncture points on the body. These run along 12 pathways or energy channels, known as meridians. Each meridian is linked to a particular organ in the body, thus each organ can be treated by stimulating the relevant meridian. In everyday practice, only about 200 acupuncture points are commonly used, stimulated by tiny needles which unblock the flow of Qi at these points. Many things, including illness and emotional states, can disturb the flow of Qi. Using needles as fine as a human hair, your acupuncturist will aim to activate your body's energy channels, treat disease, boost your immune system, promote your body's natural healing powers and alleviate fatigue.

In addition to the 12 main meridians, there are eight others, many of which are specific to women's physiology and childbirth. Of particular interest are the *ren* and *chong* channels. The *ren* channel, for example, controls conception and nourishment of the fetus and, according to the Chinese tradition, a woman can only conceive when the *ren* and *chong* channels are functioning well. The *chong* channel does not have a specific pathway but intersects the *ren* and kidney channels in places.

In Chinese medicine, harmony and balance are dependent on the smooth, uninterrupted flow of Qi. According to this philosophy, the Qi is responsible for the proper function of all spiritual, emotional, mental

The Meridians
There are 12 main meridians, or energy channels, in the body. In addition there are two important extra meridians – the *ren* and *chong* – which run down the front and back midline of the body and which are specific to women's physiology and childbirth.

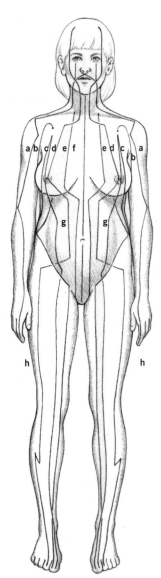

a Large intestine
b Lung
c Spleen
d Stomach
e Kidney
f Midline/Ren
g Liver
h Gall bladder

and physical processes. Although the use of needles is most commonly associated with the practice of acupuncture, a therapist may also bring elements of massage, tissue stimulation similar to that used in osteopathy, herbal medicine, dietary advice and recommendations for therapeutic exercise such as *Qi gong* into his or her practice in order to help a patient restore balance.

Although it may seem, in theory, a rather simple therapy, acupuncture involves the knowledge of a complex system of health. Your therapist will be applying aspects of Chinese medicine which include, for example, balancing the yin (female energy) and yang (male energy) in the body. He or she will also be balancing other opposing forces which form part of the philosophy of yin and yang, such as heat and cold, internal and external, deficiency and excess, as well as assessing and responding to the cyclical effect of the five elements (water, wood, fire, earth and metal, the influence of which can be felt at different times of the year) in your body.

There is probably no reason why you should concern yourself too deeply with the philosophy behind the practice if you do not want to. However, since some of these principles encompass what you eat (for instance, some foods are considered yin and others yang, and an imbalance in these foods can lead to disharmony in the body) and other aspects of your lifestyle, it may be worthwhile to go into greater depth about your treatment with your practitioner.

Acupuncture is one of the most thoroughly researched and documented of all the alternative medical practices. As such you can choose it with confidence to help a variety of conditions. In addition to treating specific problems, acupuncture has been shown to have a strengthening effect on the immune system as well as on the secretion of gastric acid and the production of red and white blood cells, and to improve circulation, blood pressure, rhythm and stroke volume of the heart. It may also stimulate a variety of hormones which help the body respond more efficiently to injury and stress.

Because it is safe and effective, with no known side-effects for mother or baby, many women (even those who feel a little nervous about the idea of needles) find acupuncture an effective way of promoting a healthy pregnancy. Although acupuncture can be applied to a wide range of disorders during pregnancy, it is most widely used for pain relief antenatally, and either to initiate labour or to relieve pain during labour. Nevertheless, acupuncture has repeatedly demonstrated its ability to gently nudge the body back into harmony, along the way relieving niggling discomforts, without causing major and unnecessary changes in body chemistry – an important consideration at any time, but especially during pregnancy.

Acupuncture in Pregnancy

The most widely acknowledged use of acupuncture in pregnancy is to correct fetal malposition, such as a baby lying in a breech or transverse position. Many studies exist to suggest that acupuncture can help as many as 7 out of 10 babies to turn into the more favourable head-down, or cephalic position. It is also a very effective way of easing minor conditions such as morning sickness. Midwife-acupuncturists report a high rate of success in treating constipation during pregnancy and it can also be useful in cases of bladder and kidney infection, aches and pains, high blood pressure, digestive disorders, skin problems and tiredness. You may find that a few general sessions with an experienced acupuncturist can do more to help maintain a healthy balance throughout your body than a few just-in-case vitamin pills from your doctor or midwife.

Acupuncture may also be useful in correcting problems of metabolism. For instance, one German study in 1994 used acupuncture to treat low iron levels in the blood. Women whose haemoglobin was on the low side of normal after giving birth were randomly given either no treatment, iron supplements or acupuncture treatment specific to the bladder, gallbladder and stomach. Blood tests after only five days of treatment confirmed that acupuncture was at least as effective as the iron supplements in helping to raise blood haemoglobin.

If you have suffered recurrent miscarriages, acupuncture may provide a way of 'relaxing' the uterine muscle, providing some protection from the possibility of miscarriage (it will not, however, prevent spontaneous abortion of a fetus which is in any way damaged).

Acupuncture may also be helpful in less direct ways. If the mother is a smoker, for example, studies exist to show that acupuncture treatment may help her kick the habit. Some acupuncturists also claim amazing results when treating breathing disorders such as asthma. If you are asthmatic and concerned that the medication you are taking may be harmful for your baby, you might consider consulting an acupuncturist.

Treatment may enable you to reduce the amount of medication you are taking.

ACUPUNCTURE IN LABOUR

Acupuncture can be used to stimulate labour and has been shown to be an effective form of pain relief during labour. There is evidence to suggest that acupuncture can cut the length of labour by up to two hours, which makes it marginally more effective than conventional forms of induction.

Unlike drug-induced induction, there have been no reported adverse effects from the use of acupuncture. What is more, the contractions stimulated by acupuncture appear to resemble those which occur when labour starts spontaneously. This is because they stimulate the release of the body's own 'labour' hormones, oxytocin and endorphins. The down side is that it can take several treatments to stimulate labour, often over a period of days. Nevertheless this inconvenience may be made up for by its demonstrated benefits over drugs.

If you are 'overdue,' that is, if you have gone more than two weeks past your due date, you might consider using acupuncture to help move things along. Only a very few midwives are qualified in the use of acupuncture. Be aware that if you are planning a hospital birth you are unlikely to be given the opportunity to bring a private practitioner along with you. Instead, have your practitioner show your birth partner some useful places to stimulate with acupressure (*see* chapter 19) in case you need help keeping your contractions going once in the delivery room.

To relieve pain in labour an acupuncturist will often use points located in your ear. Once the needles are in place, you will be able to move around freely and take up any position which feels comfortable during labour. Because production of the body's own pain-killing hormones is being stimulated, some women are even able to fall asleep during contractions. Occasionally a practitioner will opt to stimulate the needles with low-frequency electricity, known as electro-acupuncture. Rather like the TENS machine, when using electro-acupuncture the mother is in control of the intensity of the stimulation, but the frequency is pre-set by the practitioner. Acupuncture is likely to be most useful in the first stage of labour and its usefulness as an analgesic tends to diminish as transition approaches. The degree of pain relief may also vary from individual to individual.

It would be misleading to say that all studies show that acupuncture reduces the length of labour. However, length of labour is not always the best measurement of success. A long labour in which the woman feels comfortable and supported is unlikely to be as stressful as a short labour in which the woman is frightened and in great pain. Many studies show that women receiving acupuncture report feeling calm, a sense of well-being and the feeling of being in control of their own labour and delivery.

TURNING A BREECH

While there is nothing inherently abnormal about a baby in a breech position, studies have shown that mothers with breeches tend to be on the receiving end of more unnecessary caesarean operations. The majority of breeches turn spontaneously before term, although a few will persist into labour. For a woman wanting a low-tech birth, being told her baby is in a breech position can be heartbreaking, bringing with it the fear of ending up with a completely medically managed labour and the belief that there must be something wrong or some danger associated with having a baby in an unusual position. Neither is particularly true.

In truth most doctors and midwives will insist on breech babies being delivered by caesarean because they have lost the skill of delivering breech babies vaginally. Delivered vaginally by an unskilled practitioner, a breech baby may be at risk from damage to the head, spinal cord and related organs from too swift or forceful a delivery. Delivered too slowly, the baby may be deprived of oxygen.

There has been a great deal of research into how acupuncture might assist the turning of a breech baby. A well-crafted study in 1999 published in the *Journal of the American Medical Association*, looked at the practice of moxibustion (or gently heating a point on the little toe, to stimulate acupuncture point bladder 67, or 'zhiyin').

In this trial, over a two-week period, 75 per cent of the babies in the moxibustion group had turned, compared to only 47 per cent in those who had no treatment. The authors believed that stimulating the zhiyin point increased fetal activity and thus the possibility of the baby turning into a more favourable position.

To turn a breech you may need a course of up to ten treatments. However, not all of these will require a visit to your therapist. During the first treatment, your practitioner will usually show you how and where to apply the heat which will carry the Qi along the urinary/bladder channel to the uterus, where it will hopefully stimulate the baby into action.

If the baby doesn't turn, don't panic. There is absolutely no reason why you shouldn't consider going ahead with a normal, low-tech birth if this is what you wish. The chances of achieving a vaginal delivery are high. Also, the evidence is very clear that the outcome for breech babies born vaginally, with the help of an experienced practitioner, is little different to the head-down variety, in other words they are not at increased risk of trauma, death or illness after birth. Seek the help of a midwife who is experienced at delivering breech babies to ensure that you and your baby get the best possible care.

WHAT TO EXPECT

In acupuncture, diagnosis is a blend of intuition and science which some Westerners, who are new to the concept, may find difficult to grasp. In fact, it's not very different from the way the average general practitioner works – making a diagnosis on the basis of an educated guess according to the symptoms you present. The critical difference is that your acupuncturist will be trying to identify a whole pattern of disturbance, rather than just reacting to your symptoms.

The number of consultations you will require will vary enormously according to the condition being treated. The average appointment lasts anywhere from 30 minutes to an hour. However, your first appointment will need to be longer because of the time needed to take a comprehensive case history. Your acupuncturist will need detailed information about your lifestyle, diet, work, medical history and emotional state. His or her diagnosis will be made on the basis of this information as well as from examination of your pulses and your tongue.

Some people feel apprehensive that the needles will hurt; in fact, acupuncture is a virtually painless process. The needles are very fine and usually only penetrate the superficial layers of skin. Because your practitioner is working with energy channels, the place where the needles are inserted may not correspond to where you are experiencing pain. Once inserted you may feel a mild, tingling sensation but as the energy flow improves you should also feel a growing sense of well-being. The needles may be removed after a minute or two or left in for up to 30 minutes. There is no pain on removal.

Your therapist may use a variety of techniques to stimulate acupuncture points, including finger pressure, massage, electricity and heat (known as moxibustion). In moxibustion, a cigar-shaped bundle of herbs known as moxa (the Chinese word for mugwort) is lit and held a short distance from the skin in order to heat either the needle or the acupoint. This should not produce any burning, though you will feel the heat.

During pregnancy, practitioners of traditional Chinese medicine also place a great deal of emphasis on the blood because of the demands of nourishing the fetus and providing milk after birth. This may lead a practitioner to make dietary recommendations in addition to any acupuncture used.

TAKE CARE

There are very few documented adverse effects from acupuncture treatment. You should make sure you go to a qualified therapist, preferably one who is used to working with pregnant women, as there are certain acupuncture points which should not be stimulated during pregnancy. A good acupuncturist will usually be cautious about over-stimulating the body during pregnancy and will generally opt for gently strengthening the body and giving advice on diet and lifestyle.

CHAPTER 10

AROMATHERAPY

NERVOUS EXHAUSTION

RESPIRATORY PROBLEMS

HIGH BLOOD PRESSURE

INSOMNIA

MORNING SICKNESS

NAUSEA

FLUID RETENTION

CYSTITIS

VAGINAL INFECTIONS

VARICOSE VEINS

SKIN PROBLEMS

PAIN RELIEF

PERINEAL PAIN

☑ **Some conditions will require a professional therapist**

☑ **Some conditions are suitable for simple self-treatment**

Smell is the most ancient of all the human senses ...

It affects our lives and emotions in ways which scientists have not even begun to fathom. Certain smells can stimulate, others can relax or invigorate. When you are pregnant your sense of smell becomes even more acute and your ability to tolerate some smells may even be lowered. You may find that scents which once made you feel good now make you nauseous and those that once lifted your spirits now make you anxious and irritable. This is a good example of how profoundly our sense of smell affects us, causing subtle and not so subtle changes in the body and the mind.

Throughout history volatile oils extracted from flowers, herbs and animal sources have been used to calm or stimulate the emotions and enhance well-being. The use of balms, ointments and scented oils is even documented in the Bible. Scent has historically been thought to have the power to heal and repel evil and as such has played a part in religious rituals across many cultures. For the Egyptians it was part of the burial ritual and a symbol of status. The Greeks believed fragrance connected them to the gods. The Romans used perfumes for seduction and herbs as aphrodisiacs, whereas in the Middle Ages perfume was used mainly to cover up the stench of disease.

The modern use of essential oils as a therapy, however, began in the 1930s when a French chemist, René Maurice Gattefosse, coined the term aromatherapy. Fascinated by the benefits of lavender oil in healing his burned hand without leaving any scars, he started to investigate the healing potential of other essential oils.

During the Second World War, a French army surgeon, Dr Jean Valnet, successfully used essential oils to treat wounded soldiers and patients in a psychiatric hospital. Not long afterwards, Marguerite Maury, an Austrian beauty therapist and biochemist, elevated aromatherapy to a holistic therapy when she began prescribing essential oils as a remedy for her patients. She is also credited with establishing the modern practice of using essential oils in massage.

Today aromatherapy is something of a catch-all phrase for a wide range of healing techniques, such as massage and steam inhalation, which involve the use of highly concentrated oils derived from plants and flowers.

UNDERSTANDING OUR SENSE OF SMELL

Odour and chemical detection is vital for the survival of most living things. For animals it is essential for finding food, mating and protection. In humans, its link to basic survival has decreased as our lives have become less dependent on being able to hunt and escape predators. Nowadays, odour detection is often thought of as a sense that enhances our lives, but is not all that necessary. Nevertheless, it is the sense of smell which allows newborn babies to find their mother's breast.

Humans have the ability to distinguish between more than 10,000 different smells. But smell is a complex sense which involves much more than the detection of odour. When we breathe in an odour we are taking in a mixture of chemicals, and in recent years it has become apparent that these chemicals can affect us in many ways. Obvious examples of this are the way glue sniffing or snorting cocaine can directly affect the mind and body. But there are more subtle, though no less devastating, examples in everyday life. Because we are constantly bombarded with smells from perfumes, fabric softeners, soaps, shampoos, room fresheners and other less pleasant smells, such as exhaust fumes, our olfactory receptors are in a state of constant stimulation.

Studies have shown that inhaling fragrances can cause changes in both the circulation and the electrical activity in the brain. Fragrances are a frequent trigger of migraine headaches and some observers feel that the over-abundance of volatile, synthetic chemicals plays an important role in multiple chemical sensitivity.

Exactly how odour is perceived and processed in the brain is not well understood since it involves complicated physical and psychological pathways which can be impossible to separate. We do know that, of all the senses, smell has the most direct connection to the mind and emotions. Studies indicate that people who have lost their sense of smell often suffer from a high incidence of psychiatric problems, such as depression and anxiety. All fragrances, natural and synthetic, are able to breach the blood/brain barrier and gain direct access to the limbic system – the emotional switchboard of the brain. Fragrances can also be absorbed through the skin; the greater the emollient quality of the product you are using, as in skin creams or oils, the greater the absorbency.

What all this means is that aromatherapy works on the mind and body at the same time. For therapeutic use there are about 150 essential oils, distilled from plants, flowers, trees, bark, grasses and seeds. Each has a distinctive chemical make-up and a unique therapeutic, psychological and physiological effect. Some are antiseptic, others are antiviral, anti-inflammatory, pain-relieving, antidepressant or expectorant. They can be used, among other things, to stimulate, relax, improve digestion and eliminate excess water.

Aromatherapy is suitable for self-help and is widely used in homes, clinics and hospitals for a variety of conditions. Essential oils can be used in baths or steam inhalations, sprinkled on pillows or sheets, or used in oil burners, diffusers and vaporizers. The way an oil is used will enhance its effect on the body. For instance, massage without essential oils has long been known to improve emotional states such as anxiety and depression, as well as reducing levels of pain. Combined with correctly selected therapeutic oils, which can be inhaled and absorbed through the skin, its effect can be even more profound.

Aromatherapy in Pregnancy

In pregnancy, aromatherapy is generally used as a kind of first aid addressing specific problems such as headache or nausea. However, regular aromatherapy massage can also work to prevent such problems occurring in the first place. There is a large body of evidence to show that massage, apart from inducing feelings of well-being, also has a strengthening effect on the immune system. It also helps to tone the muscles, relieving aches and pains, particularly in the lower back. As such, a regular visit to the aromatherapist or massage by your partner could become one of the most pleasant parts of your health regime.

In addition, aromatherapy can be used to help counteract fluid retention and to relieve varicose veins. Some women swear that aromatherapy massage beginning early in pregnancy helps to prevent stretch marks. Certainly it can't hurt and for some it may genuinely help improve the elasticity of the skin.

Aromatherapy massage during pregnancy is believed to improve the elasticity of the perineum – the fleshy patch of skin between the opening of the vagina and the anus. A good base oil, such as sweet almond or apricot kernel oil, can be mixed with a very few drops of a skin-softening essential oil such as lavender. You should aim to massage your perineum, inside and out, daily from about 32 weeks. Doing so may help it stretch without tearing during the birth of your baby. If you find doing this hard because of your increasing bulk, consider asking your partner to do it for you.

AROMATHERAPY IN LABOUR

If your birth partner is not confident about his or her massage skills, now is the time to start learning. A competent massage during labour can help to ease anxiety and depression. It can also help shorten the length of labour. But the reverse is also true; an unskilled massage can leave the mother feeling as if her skin has been rubbed raw without delivering any real benefit. If you are seeing an aromatherapist, why not ask if your birth partner can come along to pick up some pointers? Some Active Birth teachers incorporate regular workshops for couples on massage during pregnancy and labour into their antenatal repertoire.

If you are near term or past your due date, self-massage is a good way to encourage labour. Nipple massage, in particular, is a good way to encourage labour in a post-dates pregnancy. In one study, the number of post-dates pregnancies was reduced by 70 per cent by this simple but effective method. By using this natural method you might avoid all the panicky medical measures which are often used on women who have gone more than a week past their expected date of delivery.

The largest study ever done into the use of aromatheraphy in labour showed that the use of essential oils can ease labour pain and shorten its duration by helping to promote relaxation. A research team in Oxford, England, studied 8,000 women for a period of eight years. They found that among those who used aromatherapy in labour there were fewer inductions and fewer caesareans, and an almost 30 per cent drop in the use of pain-relieving drugs.

During labour, women use essential oils in a variety of ways. Often they are used in oil burners, diffusers or on light-bulbs to enhance the quality of the atmosphere in the room. A good, portable way to give yourself a quick pick-me-up in labour is to sprinkle your favourite oil on a hanky and inhale from this as needed.

Even after birth, essential oils continue to be useful. Adding lavender oil to your bath can significantly reduce perineal trauma and pain. If you are finding it uncomfortable to urinate after birth, keep a small jug of water containing a dilute solution of lavender near the toilet. Pour this over your genital area as you urinate and it will ease the stinging as well as aid the healing of any tears or stitches.

USING ESSENTIAL OILS

Essential oils are a simple, portable way of taking care of yourself. There are endless ways of using them, the most common of which are:

In the bath   Mix your choice of essential oil or oils in a light carrier, such as apricot kernel oil, or in a neutral, water-dispersing oil which you can purchase at some health food shops and natural toiletry stores. Alternatively, mix it into a small amount of whole milk. Pour this mixture into the bath. If possible, aim to relax in the bath for at least 15 minutes.

For massage   A good way of addressing skin problems, aching muscles and joints, fluid retention and for preventing stretch marks. Always use essential oils diluted in a light carrier oil. When massaging the belly, use a light, clockwise motion.

As a compress   This method is good for bruises, headaches, varicose veins, burns and scalds. Add between eight and ten drops of essential oil to half a cup of water. Disperse well. Soak a face cloth in the mixture and apply to the relevant part of the body.

As an inhalation   A particularly good choice if you have a cold, cough or any other breathing difficulty. A simple and portable way to make an inhalation is to put a few drops of your chosen oil on a hanky. Wrap this in a plastic bag and carry it with you to use as and when you need to. At home, you can make a steam inhalation using a bowl of hot water and five to ten drops of essential oil. Lean over the bowl with a towel over your head and breathe deeply. Alternatively, you can now buy hand-held inhalers, which are small plastic containers, not unlike coffee mugs, with a special mask which attaches to the top.

In foot baths   Fill a basin large enough to take both of your feet with hand-hot water. Then add eight to ten drops of your favourite oil. This is a good way to soothe feet after a long day. If your ankles are swollen, try following the hot bath with a cool one to improve circulation. You can do the same thing for sore, swollen hands.

As room scents   You can spread the scent of an essential oil throughout a room using an oil burner, or by placing one or two drops on a cool light-bulb before turning the light on. If you heat your home with radiators, place five drops of essential oil in a bowl containing a little water and place this on top of the radiator.

Almost anyone can become quickly competent at choosing and mixing their own unique blends of essential oils. There are, however, certain basic guidelines you should follow:

• Never take essential oils orally.

• Always store your oils in a dark-blue or brown bottle in a cool place. When you are not using them make sure the bottle top is tightly sealed. Jasmine and citrus oils may last better if stored in a refrigerator.

• Once opened, most oils will keep their therapeutic properties for up to two years. But some, especially citrus oils, lose their potency after around six months.

• Don't store essential oils near homeopathic remedies – even with the bottle tops on they can potentially inactivate the homeopathic remedies.

• Don't administer any oil for more than three weeks without a break. The olfactory receptors can literally become exhausted, at which point the therapeutic value of the oil is lost. Depending on how often and how strongly you use them, this rule can also apply to room scents.

• You get what you pay for. Oils from readily available sources which are easy to extract the oil from, such as oranges, are relatively cheap. But oils from rare sources or those where the process of extracting oil is difficult, such as jasmine and rose, will always be expensive. Cheaper oils are either synthetic or cut with other less expensive oils. Jasmine, for instance, may be mixed with ylang ylang and rose may be mixed with geranium, bois de rose or palmarosa. Adulterated oils will not have the same therapeutic effect as pure oils.

• Only a very few essential oils are safe to use neat on the skin. The best way to use most oils is to mix them in a base, or carrier, oil. Simple sunflower oil from your kitchen cupboard is as good a choice as any. Other good choices include sweet almond, apricot kernel, grapeseed, safflower and hazelnut oils. To enrich a base oil, try adding heavier oils such as carrot, borage seed, avocado, evening primrose oil, jojoba, wheatgerm or sesame oils. Because they are so rich and heavy, these oils should account for not more than 10 per cent of any base mixture.

• When mixing oils in a base, there is a general rule which says you should use no more than 1 drop of essential oil to 1 millilitre. For example, a tablespoon of oil equals about 15ml – thus you could use up to 15 drops. However, during pregnancy when your sense of smell is greatly heightened you can use less and still gain the same results; 1 drop of essential oil to every 2ml of base oil should be sufficient. After birth, if you are considering using massage for your baby, the mixture should be even more dilute. Before embarking on baby aromatherapy massage consider consulting a professional practitioner to make sure you are not overwhelming your baby's sensitive system with fragrance.

• When you are mixing essential oils, try to keep it simple – no more than five different oils in a single mixture.

• If you have very sensitive skin do a patch test first. Mix two or three drops of essential oil in a tablespoon of base oil. Put some of this mixture on to a fabric plaster and leave this on the inside of your arm for 24 hours or until any irritation occurs.

Is it 'Natural'?

Today, everybody is jumping on the aromatherapy bandwagon. But while there are a number of 'aromatherapy' products available in supermarkets and chemists, many of the fragrances used in them are synthetic. Artificial fragrances can be found in bath oils, shampoos, lip balms and body rubs. They are also becoming more common in dish detergent, fabric softeners and other household cleaners. They are also used in foods, where they are called flavours or aromas.

The cosmetic industry long ago abandoned the use of genuinely natural ingredients. Today it bases its products on fragrances derived from petrochemicals. Synthetic oils, however, do not work in the same way as natural ones and may produce a range of undesired effects. Several bath preparations, in particular, say they contain 'natural' ingredients such as citrus or lavender. What they really mean is that they contain synthetic fragrances which are 'nature identical'.

Studies have shown that inhaling synthetic fragrance chemicals can cause negative circulatory changes in the brain. Subtle negative changes in brainwave activity can also occur with exposure to petrochemical fragrances. Perhaps not surprisingly, these types of fragrances are a frequent trigger of migraine headaches.

To produce the desired results, essential oils should always be from natural sources. When you are buying any essential oil or fragranced product, assure yourself that it is from a natural source by looking for the Latin name of the flower or herb on the label. Otherwise you could be buying a synthetic oil or an adulterated mixture derived from petrochemicals.

WHAT TO EXPECT

Like any other competent therapist, your aromatherapist should take a complete case history at your first session. The therapist will choose a mixture of oils specifically for you, depending on what was uncovered during the history-taking. Most aromatherapists use massage to enhance the effect of the essential oil, so you may be asked to undress and lie down, covered with a warm towel or sheet, on the massage couch or table. They may employ a number of different massage techniques, including shiatsu or reflexology. The depth of the massage and the parts of the body massaged will be chosen to suit your needs and comfort. An aromatherapy massage should never hurt.

Your aromatherapist should be qualified to treat a wide range of health conditions. Make sure you are not going to someone who is simply trained to use aromatherapy as a beauty treatment or for general relaxation. Such therapists generally have only completed short courses in aromatherapy and may not have the training necessary to ensure the health and well-being of a pregnant woman. If you are unsure about your therapist's credentials, ask.

To find a qualified aromatherapist, contact the International Federation of Aromatherapists or the International Society of Professional Aromatherapists (ISPA).

TAKE CARE

There is ongoing disagreement, even among professional aromatherapists, concerning which oils are safe during pregnancy and which are not and new research is coming in all the time. For instance, recent trials in France suggest that, contrary to traditional thought, eucalyptus is safe to use in pregnancy. In everyday use, most essential oils are used in such small quantities by women that the risks are little more than theoretical. Such cautions may be most relevant for women who have trouble conceiving or who have a history of miscarriage. Even so, some may reason that it is better to err on the side of caution. If your aromatherapist makes a blend specially for you or uses a unique blend for general massage, always ask for a list of ingredients.

Even if an oil is not specifically contraindicated during pregnancy, it may have an unwanted effect on you. Skin irritations are not uncommon; bergamot and other oils in the citrus family, for instance, can increase the photosensitivity of the skin, and should not be used if your skin is going to be directly exposed to the sun. Perhaps more importantly, certain oils can have an effect on blood pressure which for some women may not be entirely therapeutic. Oils such as rosemary, sage, hyssop and black pepper can raise blood pressure, while others such as lavender, clary sage and ylang ylang can lower it dramatically. If you are allergic to chrysanthemums, asters, marigold, goldenrod or ragweed, you may also be allergic to camomile.

Women who have allergies to nuts may experience a skin reaction to some base oils such as almond or peanut oil. If this applies to you, make sure you double-check which oil your therapist is using.

The following oils are considered unsuitable for use during pregnancy:
Emenagogues – can stimulate uterine bleeding

Basil	Lemon Balm
Camphor	Marjoram
Clary Sage*	Myrrh
Cypress	Nutmeg
Hyssop	Peppermint*
Jasmine*	Rose*
Juniper	Rosemary
Lavender*	Sage

Abortifacients – can stimulate labour and can cause miscarriage

Mugwort	Savin
Pennyroyal	Tansy
Plecanthrus	Thuja
Rue	Wormwood
Sage	

*Most women can use these oils during pregnancy without any problems. However, those who are prone to miscarriage should exercise caution and wait until the second trimester before using them. Side-effects are unlikely but if any should occur, discontinue use. See the chart on page 157 for a range of essential oils for pregnancy and birth, a basic selection of oils to ease a wide range of conditions.

DO IT YOURSELF

You can make a relaxing, aromatic bath by choosing one, or a combination of two or three essential oils. Add a total of four to six drops to 5ml of base oil. The reason for using a base oil is that oil does not disperse fully in water. Mixing it in a carrier will ensure that your skin does not come into contact with undiluted oil, which can cause skin reactions in some women. You can then pour some of the mixture directly into your bath. Try choosing from the following herbs:

Camomile, mandarin, lavender, lemongrass, sandalwood, geranium, rose, jasmine, ylang-ylang, lemon, bergamot, orange, rosewood and neroli.

AROMATHERAPY IN YOUR KITCHEN

One good way to stimulate your senses and nourish your body at the same time is to expand the concept of aromatherapy to include the foods that you cook and eat. Many of the herbs we use for medicinal purposes are also foods. Given the choice between taking a medicine made from herbs and eating a good meal with therapeutic herbs, many would choose the more natural and enjoyable route of a meal. You may also find that using natural aromatics in this way makes cooking a more relaxing and enjoyable experience.

Fresh and flavourful food is one of life's great pleasures. Almost any food can have an 'aromatherapeutic' effect. Think of how you feel when you smell fresh coffee being brewed, the lift you get from smelling the zest of a lemon, the way apple pie or vanilla can take you back to your childhood or how chestnuts roasting on an open fire signal winter and Christmas.

The smell of our food is inexorably linked to our enjoyment of it. In fact, taste and smell are the two most directly linked of our senses. When you have a cold and your nose is blocked up, nothing tastes the same because you cannot smell it. Aroma is the essence of food, but as well as making food taste good, it can also enhance our sense of well-being.

Herbs and spices used in culinary quantities will not act as particularly strong medicine, which is why you can include some seasonings in your food that you could not use as an essential oil or even a herbal preparation. Instead, they are a pleasant adjunct to any other therapies you may be having. Consider the therapeutic properties of the following herbs and spices, chosen for their reputed effect on the female reproductive system. If you have been previously shy about using seasoning, now might be a good time to experiment.

Healthy Herbs

Herbs will add subtle flavours to almost any dish. Always use the fresh herb and tear, don't cut the leaves. Gently crushing the leaves by scrunching them up in your hand or lightly bruising them using a mortar and pestle is a good way of releasing their aromas.

Basil fortifies the digestive and nervous systems and can be a good remedy for headaches and insomnia. It is also a good diuretic. When using it in cooking, opt for the fresh leaves and wait until the very last moment before adding them to your dish. Try scattering it on tomato salads, in soups and to egg, rice and mushroom dishes. Make your own pesto sauce, or put some fresh leaves into olive oil for a pungent salad dressing (don't worry if the leaves turn black).

Dill has a sharp/sweet taste, somewhere between mint and aniseed. It is a natural bactericide, diuretic and digestive soother and can be effective against cystitis and other bladder infections. Use it liberally with seafood, especially salmon. Sprinkle it onto salads or lightly steamed vegetables, especially new or baked potatoes. You can also add the seeds to stews, soups or as a topping on cooked vegetables or in rice dishes.

Fennel is a relative of dill and has a slightly milder flavour. Its traditional uses are for lack of appetite, poor digestion, fatigue, fluid retention, headaches and bladder infections. It is also helpful in cases of anaemia. Fennel is best used with fish but is equally appetizing in a range of fresh salads. As an alternative, put the seeds into a pepper mill and grind over meats, pulse dishes or fish.

Hyssop should **only** ever be taken as a fresh herb since the essential oil can be toxic, even fatal. Flowers and young tops are good for colds, coughs, flu, asthma and bronchitis. Sprinkle the leaves in salads, or mix chopped leaves into soft cheese, butter, sauces or dips. Used with meat and game, it acts as a counterbalance for the fattiness of the meal.

Lemon Balm is very useful for emotional states such as depression and anxiety. It can also ease the symptoms of stress, such as headache, migraine and insomnia. The essential oil is not safe to use during pregnancy as it can cause uterine bleeding, but in the kitchen you can safely use the fresh leaves in (non-alcoholic) cocktails, in stuffings and in both savoury and fruit salads. It goes well with fish and can be infused in milk for a lemony milk pudding.

Mint is a sedative and is good for the nervous system. It is an effective blood cleanser and has antiseptic and antibacterial properties. Mint is the traditional sauce for lamb but has many other uses. Put it in tall cool drinks in the summer. Mix it with bulgar wheat for a delicious salad.

Sprinkle over new potatoes or peas or use in salads or dressings. It is also delicious mixed in with chutneys or yoghurts as a cooling accompaniment to spicy foods, such as curries.

Parsley has numerous uses, including as a blood purifier, general tonic, diuretic and digestive aid. It is an effective treatment for constipation and the French revere it in much the same way that the Chinese revere ginseng. Don't just plop it on the side of your plate as in a third rate café. Stir it into omelettes, vegetable and rice dishes. Mix it with some butter, spread this on some crusty bread and bake briefly for a quick snack. Add it to mashed potato and use it when making fish or meat balls.

Sage is an ancient remedy used to normalize the female reproductive system. Eaten raw it can also be effective in rheumatic conditions, catarrh and excessive sweating. A relative of common sage, Clary Sage can be used to treat fatigue, depression, headaches and sore throats. Add to salads, soups and stuffings for rich meats like pork and goose. Make a seasoning by grinding up dried sage leaves with coarse sea salt. This can be used on almost any savoury dish. Alternatively, make a uniquely flavoured honey by adding freshly dried sage leaves. This can then be used in herbal teas and sweet dishes to give them a therapeutic boost.

Tarragon can settle the stomach and relieve constipation. It can clear the body of intestinal parasites, ease fluid retention and improve the appetite. Because it is so savoury you may not need to use as much salt in cooked dishes – a bonus for those suffering from hypertension. Its most popular use is with chicken, but it can also be used in salads and omelettes. Put some in a bottle of good-quality vinegar for a tasty condiment.

Thyme is a general tonic and an aid to digestion. It is also useful for colds, coughs, flu, asthma and sinus headaches. Some sources claim it also acts as an antioxidant. Thyme is best used fresh in marinades and sauces, stocks and stuffings. It is a staple of slow-cooked casseroles and stews and is reputed to 'fix' the iron in meat as well as making it more digestible. Crushed leaves make excellent herb oils and vinegars.

Special Spices

Spices generally add a more pungent taste to foods. Wherever possible, it is best to buy the whole spice and grind or crush it yourself. This way the aroma will be stronger and you will benefit from more of the active ingredients.

Aniseed can be used to combat nervous indigestion and palpitations. It is also effective against flatulence, hiccups and fluid retention. The seeds go particularly well with figs. Use them also with fish and in vegetable dishes, soups and curries. The fresh leaves can be added to salads or at the last minute to steamed vegetables.

Caraway has traditionally been used to make foods more digestible. It also helps combat bad breath and dyspepsia. Sprinkle fresh leaves over cabbage, potato and beetroot dishes. If you bake your own bread, particularly rye bread, add caraway seed to the mixture. Add also to soft cheeses to make an unusual sandwich spread. If you grow your own, you can also eat the tap roots as you would parsnip.

Cardamom is a good digestive stimulant and diuretic. Buy the whole green or bleached white seeds to use, lightly crushed, in rice dishes, curries and meat stews. Freshly ground cardamom can give a surprising lift to an everyday fruit salad. It can also be infused in milk to make a spicy custard or rice pudding.

Cinnamon is a first-class antiseptic and digestive aid. It freshens the breath and aids recovery from colds and flu. It is equally pleasant in savoury dishes, such as stews, stuffings, pickles and relishes, as it is in sweet dishes, such as stewed fruits and pies. It's lovely on hot buttered toast and can be used to spice up rice or milk puddings. Try using a cinnamon stick to stir hot chocolate or milky coffee.

Cumin is a good general tonic. It is antiseptic, antibacterial and is reputed to help improve circulation. It can be delicious added to the marinade for barbecues or kebabs. You can make a spicy Eastern-style salad with tomatoes, green peppers, courgettes and/or aubergines with a little powdered cumin sprinkled on top. Use the whole seeds in pickles or preserves.

Ginger can be used liberally in your cooking to combat nausea as well as being a good antiseptic. It stimulates the gastric juices and can relieve symptoms of sore throats, colds and flu. Ginger is as good on ice-cream as it is in a casserole. It is also tasty in pickles and cheese dishes and can be used effectively in all forms of baking, particularly cakes and breads.

Horseradish counters fluid retention, aids digestion and eases coughs and colds. It can be difficult, but not impossible, to buy fresh. The grated root can be mixed with cream, yoghurt or vinegar and used in sauces for meats, especially roast beef and fish.

Juniper acts as a blood cleanser and is effective in rheumatic conditions such as arthritis. It acts against bladder infections and stimulates the liver and gallbladder. The fresh berries are best lightly crushed and cooked with meat and game. Used with garlic and sea salt, they are a wonderful accompaniment for cabbage and other green vegetables. It can also be used in a variety of stuffings, sauces, marinades and pâtés.

Nutmeg can be beneficial for convalescents and those who are overtired. It acts as a stimulant, tonic and digestive. It can ease flatulence and is reportedly good for the heart. Use in milk and rice puddings, in white or cheese sauces. Liberal doses can transform mashed potatoes and other vegetable dishes. Sprinkle over hot chocolate or warm milk for a quick pick-me-up.

Peppercorns come in green, black, white and pink and are actually a fruit. Pepper is a well-known digestive and can stimulate the appetite in those who are anaemic. It can purify the blood, ease lung and bronchial infections and relieve shock and stress. Use in savoury stocks and marinades and liberally over salads and hot vegetable dishes. Coat steaks thoroughly before grilling, and add crushed peppercorns to vinegars and oils to make spicy dressings. Always buy whole peppercorns and grind as required. Pre-ground spice quickly loses its active properties.

Essential oil	How does it work?	Most useful for	Try blending With
Camomile *Matricaria chamomilla* (German) *Anthemis nobilis* (Roman)	Anti-inflammatory, antiseptic, digestive, tonic	Skin problems, wound healing, heartburn, indigestion, headache, cystitis, fluid retention, nausea, back pain, constipation, soothing and calming	Almost any other oil but particularly lavender, geranium, jasmine, bergamot, rose, neroli, clary sage, sandalwood, mandarin
Clary Sage* *Salvia sclarea*	Hypotensive, aphrodisiac, digestive, antidepressant, antiseptic, sedative, tonic	Anxiety, stress, improving circulation, relieves pain and cramp, enhances contractions	Orange, grapefruit, mandarin, geranium, sandalwood, lavender
Eucalyptus *Eucalyptus globulus*	Diuretic, expectorant, analgesic, antiseptic, stimulant	Headaches, colds and flu, cystitis, diarrhoea, muscle aches, respiratory conditions	Lavender, camomile, mandarin, tea tree, lemon
Geranium *Pelargonium odorantissimum*	Antiseptic, astringent, diuretic, refreshing, toning, hypotensive	Fluid retention, anxiety, high blood pressure, diarrhoea, tension, depression, skin conditions, cramp, varicose veins	Bergamot, clary sage, orange, rose, lavender, jasmine and sandalwood
Grapefruit *Citrus xpadadisi*	Uplifting, tonifying	Stress, exhaustion, skin conditions, constipation	Bergamot, neroli, tea tree, clary sage, sandalwood, mandarin and other citrus oils, geranium, lavender
Jasmine *Jasminum officinale*	Antidepressant, stimulant	Enhances uterine action, regulates contractions, relieves tension	Rose, sandalwood, neroli, geranium mandarin and other citrus oils, camomile, lavender
Lavender *Lavandula augustifolia* *Lavandula officinalis*	Antibacterial, decongestant, antidepressant, aids sleep, reduces pain	Skin complaints, insomnia, colds and flu, burns and scalds, anxiety and depression, cramp, muscleaches, stretch marks, back pain, heals wounds, lowers blood pressure, eases headache	Most oils but in particular, geranium, jasmine, camomile, mandarin
Mandarin (tangerine) *Citrus reticulata*	Refreshing, uplifting, antiseptic, antispasmodic, sedative, digestive and tonic	Depression, cramp, anxiety, heartburn, constipation, nausea, stretch marks	Particularly lavender and neroli, but also sandalwood, geranium, jasmine, camomile
Neroli (orange blossom) *Citrus bigaradia* *Citrus aurantium*	Antidepressant, sedative, antibacterial, digestive, tonic, aids circulation	Constipation, flatulence, diarrhoea, oedema, insomnia, stress, skin conditions, stretch marks, eases breathing during labour	Geranium, grapefruit, mandarin, lemon, sandalwood, clary sage, ylang ylang, rose, camomile
Rose *Rosa damascena* *Rosa centifolia*	Antidepressant, sedative, antiseptic, diuretic, laxative, uterine tonic	Depression, anxiety, loss of libido, enhancing contractions	Mandarin, sandalwood, neroli, camomile, jasmine, lavender, clary sage, geranium, ylang ylang
Sandalwood *Santalum album*	Antiseptic, aphrodisiac, digestive, diuretic, expectorant, sedative and tonic	Respiratory infections, skin conditions, anxiety, fluid retention, lack of energy, heartburn, varicose veins, soothes and refreshes	Ylang ylang, rose, neroli, jasmine, lavender and geranium, bergamot, tea tree
Tea Tree *Melaleuca alternifolia*	Antiseptic, antifungal, anti-inflammatory, stimulates the immune system	Cystitis, skin conditions, respiratory problems	Lavender, geranium, mandarin, lemon, grapefruit will all mask its rather medicinal smell

*Not recommended for use in early pregnancy, but can be safely used in late pregnancy and during labour

CHAPTER 11

COUNSELLING AND PSYCHOTHERAPY

WHAT IT'S BEST FOR

RELATIONSHIP PROBLEMS
IMPROVING SELF-IMAGE
CHANGING PATTERNS OF SELF-SABOTAGE
MANAGING CHANGE
CONFLICT RESOLUTION/NEGOTIATION SKILLS
DREAMWORK
OVERCOMING SEXUAL ABUSE
FACING FEELINGS OF LOSS
SUPPORT THROUGH DEPRESSION
EXPRESSING ANGER AND RESENTMENT
CHANGING INAPPROPRIATE BEHAVIOUR

☑ **Requires a professional therapist**

Most people enter therapy at pivotal points in their lives ...

A birth or death, a marriage, divorce or separation, redundancy or embarking on a new career – all these things change our lives and challenge who we are, or who we think we are. It is often at these points, when stress may be at its highest, that we discover that old habits, excuses and behaviours, built up over a lifetime, simply don't work anymore.

Pregnancy is a time when a woman may acquire a whole range of new life skills. Which skills these are depends on who she is and what kind of life she has. For some, who have lived more or less sedentary lives, it may signal a time to get fit; for those who feel that they lack emotional resources, or psychological savvy, it is often a useful time to begin the process of acquiring these.

Pregnancy and birth are a paradox. On the one hand, they are the most ordinary and universal of experiences. On the other, they are also the most extraordinary and personal of human experiences.

Early in pregnancy most women realize that pregnancy and the impending birth are more than just physical events. While many women find that their physical needs are more or less catered for during this time, their emotional needs are often dismissed as trivial. This imbalance ignores the fact that being pregnant involves a substantial shift in self-perception as well as massive changes in all our relationships and day-to-day lives.

Some women are lucky enough to have family and friends who support them through these changes. Others may feel that they need time and space to talk to someone outside their immediate circle about what they are going through, and maybe even vent 'unpopular' feelings such as anger, resentment, depression and self-doubt. This is where therapy may be useful.

When considering therapy there are two broad categories from which to choose: counselling and psychotherapy. Confusion exists about the difference between the two, and for some individual practitioners the distinction is also beginning to disappear. In general, counsellors are problem-solvers specializing in one specific area such as bereavement, addiction, abuse, marital problems and, more recently, birth. A counselling session generally deals with the here and now, helping the person to find immediate solutions. Only occasionally will it delve more deeply into the root causes of those problems or assist clients in making long-term changes in their behaviour.

Psychotherapists are trained to provide a context in which the individual can explore their emotional responses, anxieties, patterns of behaviour, individual potential and limitations, in some depth. Psychotherapy involves establishing a 'safe' relationship with your therapist and a regular routine of sessions which support that relationship. Over the course of therapy the individual is helped to express thoughts and feelings which have been long suppressed. She is also encouraged to make connections between the present and the past in order to better face the future. Inappropriate and ineffective behaviour will also be challenged, with a view to creating more effective ways of meeting needs and expressing feelings.

Perhaps because of the need to talk things out, and the value which they place on interpersonal communication, more women than men tend to take up the option of seeing a counsellor or therapist. This and the influence of many powerful female analysts has changed the face of therapy in recent times. During the latter half of the twentieth century psychotherapy, in particular, has benefited from the influence of feminism. What was once a masculine, rational, aloof process has now become more of a holistic, client-centred one where the influence of all aspects of a person's life are taken into account.

BEING IN CONTROL

Therapy is seen by some as a way to gain a sense of control over their lives. They believe the Western ideal that 'taking control' of life is an achievable and necessary goal. Therapy often exposes this ideal for what it largely is – the mere illusion of control. The paradox of therapy is that it often teaches control by first exploring those things which we cannot control.

In reality, there are only two things which are genuinely within your control: 1) the way you perceive yourself and 2) the way you behave.

When you become a mother you will also briefly have some control over your children. You will have control over what you teach them, how they behave and how they feel about themselves. But often these things are simply a reflection of your relationship with yourself and with the world.

Therapy is a way of shining a light on those things which are within your control as well as those things which are not. Once this happens, it is often easier to stop trying to control everyone and everything around you. It is also easier to stop taking responsibility for things which are simply outside your control.

For some, therapy provides a form of 'mothering', with the therapist taking on the symbolic role of the 'good' mother. This is not just crass symbolism but a response to a deep need in many of us to feel connected. Our first experience of connectedness is with our mothers and being able to return to this state means being able to return to a place where we felt whole. Having reconnected with this experience, many individuals feel able to face the future with a more confident outlook. For women in particular, therapy can become a way to reconnect with the powerful aspects of childbearing and childrearing; a chance to celebrate, not denigrate, their femaleness.

When a women is pregnant she undergoes some powerful psychological changes. Most of us don't have a clue about what these entail until it's our turn, but common experiences include discovering a wide range of emotions and the humbling reality that you are not as clear-thinking or highly evolved as you believed yourself to be. Pregnancy also challenges the woman to relinquish and redefine her ideas about control. Such feelings can bring up profound insecurities which may be best met with the help of a qualified therapist.

THERAPY IN PREGNANCY

During pregnancy, therapy can be invaluable in helping you to meet fears and anxieties, clear past experiences, come to terms with yourself and even prevent depression from occurring after birth. We now examine some of the reasons why women seek the help of a therapist at this time.

Overcoming a Difficult Birth

For some women a second pregnancy can be even more anxiety-provoking than the first. If the first pregnancy was medically directed, if something went wrong as a result of medical interference, or if the woman has a history of miscarriage or stillbirth, the thought of going through it all again can bring up feelings of extreme apprehension and doubt.

Second-time mothers who have been unable to work through a disappointing or traumatic birth experience, bring to the next birth all the baggage of the first. Often when such a woman chooses to seek the help of a therapist, she is doing so for very positive reasons. For instance, she may recognize that the last experience left her very traumatized and unable to move forward physically or emotionally until she begins to clear the past. Or she may recognize that she may have had a role to play in allowing others to take over responsibility for the process from her. It is probably important that such a woman finds a therapist with experience of dealing with pregnancy or birth. Rigid attitudes about how and where women should give birth and what they are 'allowed' to feel upset about in this regard persist even among supposedly liberal therapists.

Past Sexual Abuse

If current estimates are correct and one in three women has suffered some form of sexual abuse as a child, then it is small wonder that so many women find pregnancy and birth so frightening. How can so many women have been abused? The answer is that abuse is more than a physical act. When we think of abuse we tend to think the worst – grown men repeatedly physically abusing young girls. But a woman can be traumatized by a single incident which happened at a crucial time of her development. The abuse may be (and usually is) physical, but at heart it is also a betrayal of trust. Such an experience can make a woman despise her body, devalue her sexuality and be very fearful about bringing a child, who may suffer the same misfortune, into this world.

A woman who has been sexually abused as a child has special and legitimate needs during pregnancy. Left unsupported through this time – when terrifying memories may surface – the prospect of labour may overwhelm her. The antenatal routine, with its focus on poking and prodding the woman, may re-enact past abuses. She may suffer in silence, fearing that telling her midwife will single her out as some sort of freak or neurotic. Or she may waver between attending antenatal clinics which make her feel more violated, and not attending at all and risking isolating herself further in her fears. For such a woman, pregnancy can be anything but joyful.

Most doctors and midwives have no counselling or therapeutic skills at all and are simply not equipped to deal with survivors of sexual abuse. If you are a survivor of incest or abuse you are much better off seeking the help of a sympathetic counsellor, with whom you can share your experiences and feelings. Seeking therapy is the first step towards valuing yourself again.

Depression

For many the experience of depression is nothing more than yesterday's bad mood. For others it is a debilitating, chronic illness which affects them and those around them. A 'bad mood' becomes a major health problem when it is severe enough and persistent enough to interfere with work, friendships, family life and even physical health. An episode of severe depression can last for several weeks or several years, and New Age definitions of depression such as 'having nowhere to put your love' deny the genuine depth of symptoms such as misery, despair, guilt and a feeling of total worthlessness.

Pregnancy and birth do not automatically increase a woman's chance of becoming depressed. A tendency towards depression may be the result of a combination of things: a family trait, nutritional imbalances, childhood losses, adult disappointments, and immediate social conditions, the combination of which will vary in each individual. In women, depression is often a secondary symptom masking other less socially acceptable feelings. It is interesting to note that rates of depression in women roughly equal rates of violent behaviour in men – and that both can be outward expressions of anger and frustration. How these feelings are expressed is mediated by what society dictates is appropriate behaviour for each sex.

Depression is an emotional state which both practitioners and patients sometimes have to 'feel' their way through, but hidden among the dark feelings of depression is often a useful design for life change.

Relationship Difficulties

The majority of women and their partners tend to muddle through relationship difficulties at this time. But for some couples, pregnancy can take the relationship to breaking point. There is a wide variety of help available for individuals and couples to support them as their relationship begins to respond to the inevitable changes which parenthood brings.

It is unlikely that pregnancy is the real cause of any marital difficulties. More often, it is simply the catalyst which brings long-standing problems into sharper focus. If you and your partner have trouble communicating with each other, therapy can help you develop better communication skills. If you can't make sense of your feelings about each other or the baby, therapy can also provide a context in which to begin to sort it out. In truth, it is usually the woman who first seeks the help of a therapist – often her partner is not very enthusiastic about the idea. But since many men feel that their needs are not being met while their wives are pregnant, the experience of seeing a therapist can prove surprisingly helpful for the man as well as his partner.

What to Expect

There are many (perhaps too many) types of therapy available. You may need to conduct some serious research before you choose which one suits you. All therapies require a time commitment. Sessions are usually weekly (though they can be more, or less, frequent) and last between 45 and 60 minutes. Unless you have very strong feelings after the first meeting that this is the wrong therapist or therapy for you, you should be willing to commit to at least six to eight sessions before you can decide whether this particular person and therapy will suit you.

Counselling

This type of therapy tends to be informal and does not usually require such a long-term time commitment. During an hour-long session, you will be encouraged to express what is on your mind that day or what has been occurring during the week, and your counsellor will make helpful suggestions. The term 'counselling' covers a wide range of approaches which can range from simple advice-giving all the way to sessions which are near indistinguishable from psychotherapy. When used as a therapy, counselling is usually associated with the work of therapist Carl Rogers, who coined the phrase 'client-centred therapy'. In such therapy, the counsellor does not interpret what is said. Instead, he or she is trained to listen attentively and empathetically to the client and reflect back, paraphrased, what he or she hears. The process of repetition and paraphrase can be helpful in clarifying day-to-day problems the client is experiencing.

Some alternative practitioners from other disciplines, such as aromatherapy and homeopathy, incorporate simple counselling skills in their practice. Because the term 'counselling' is so broad, it is best to ask the therapist what approach he or she takes, how their sessions usually progress and what kind of training they have had.

You can get a list of counsellors in your area from the British Association for Counselling (*see* page 297).

Psychotherapy

Different psychotherapists practise in different ways and require different things from their clients. Therapists with Freudian or Kleinian backgrounds usually prefer their clients to lie down facing away from them. Jungian therapists prefer to sit across or at an angle from their clients. Still others give clients the freedom to choose how they wish to position themselves during a session. A psychotherapeutic session usually lasts 50 minutes to an hour.

A psychotherapist is not there to hand solutions to you and psychotherapy usually requires a long-term commitment in order to see real change. Most therapists maintain what is known as a 'mindful presence'; listening attentively to what you are saying, offering insights when it seems appropriate, but always referring the problem back to you for discussion and exploration. Some will use a variety of techniques to help you gain insight into your situation. This may include dreamwork, breathing, bodywork, guided imagination and play-acting.

To find a psychotherapist in your local area, contact the United Kingdom Council for Psychotherapy (*see* page 302).

REBIRTHING

Birth is the 'original experience' for each of us. Rebirthing, what is known as a regression technique, provides a way of reliving that original experience. The eminent French doctor, Frederick LeBoyer, suggested many years ago that birth can be painful and traumatic for the baby, though this is probably more true of high-tech, high-intervention births. The experience of a painful or traumatic birth could, LeBoyer suggested, affect the child's outlook on life, leaving it with a very negative perception

What Stops Us from Growing?

There's an analogy which a prominent Jungian analyst uses to illustrate why so many of us get 'stuck' in our lives. She would say that if someone who can't change a light-bulb is drawn to someone who can, that might be considered a 'good fit'. After all, she's found someone to complete her, to fill in the gaps, to do for her the things which she finds so difficult. But she may also find herself in a stagnant situation where she will never have the chance of learning how to change a light-bulb. In fact it's probably a relationship where neither party can grow because they're so locked into their roles of 'light-bulb-changer' and 'not-light-bulb-changer'.

Our ability to change and grow is always there, but it is often hidden away deep inside of us. Much of our potential to change never gets a chance to surface because humans can be very lazy creatures, much more willing to accept our so-called limitations, and to have fantasies of being able, rather than having to face the possibility of disappointment when we try.

of the world. Rebirthers believe that if a person can be helped to relive their own birth experience in a positive way, that person's outlook on life and their experience of life from that point can become more positive.

There are two different types of rebirthing, both originating from America: one was devised by Leonard Orr, the other by Frank Lake.

Orr's rebirthing employs a breathing exercise. The therapist and client sit in a quiet room, pillows and blankets may be used to cover the client if necessary. The client will be asked to breathe in and out in a regular way. Usually this goes on for an hour or so until the client experiences a feeling of 'release' – the eventual aim of rebirthing. However, the client and therapist can also agree a maximum time limit for the breathing exercise to limit the strain on the client.

Orr's method also employs affirmations, or positive statements which are repeated over and over again. The affirmation is often tailored to the individual's needs but typically is something like, 'Every breath increases my aliveness', or 'I feel great love for people'. Sometimes the rebirthing takes place under water, since this is closer to the original fetal environment. With this variation on Orr's therapy, a snorkel is used to help the person remain underwater for a long time.

Frank Lake's rebirthing process takes place in a group setting. One member chooses to be reborn and lies on the floor. The other members physically assemble themselves into a simulated womb which surrounds the rebirther. There is liberal use of cushions which act as buffers between the group/womb and the rebirther/fetus. In order to simulate the growth of the fetus in the contained environment, group members gradually apply increasing pressure, usually by sitting, lying or pressing in on the fetal member. The fetus decides, usually when overcome by claustrophobia, when it is time to come out. This can be a physically and emotionally demanding experience. However, if done with sensitivity it can also be rewarding.

These regression techniques are very different from each other so if you are interested in rebirthing, make sure you know which one you are signing up for. Centres offering rebirthing are listed at the back of this book.

CHAPTER 12

HERBS AND FLOWER REMEDIES

WHAT IT'S BEST FOR

ANAEMIA
CRAMP
HEARTBURN
CONSTIPATION
CYSTITIS
FLUID RETENTION
HAEMORRHOIDS
INSOMNIA
HIGH BLOOD PRESSURE
THREATENED MISCARRIAGE
INFECTIONS
EXHAUSTION IN LABOUR
PERINEAL CARE
MOOD CHANGES

☑ **Some conditions require a professional therapist**
☑ **Some conditions are suitable for simple self-treatment**

Before books, before 'experts' there were medicinal plants …

Herbal remedies are part of a tradition which stretches back long before our first human ancestors. Animals instinctively turn to certain plants when they are ill, and perhaps watching these other animals is how humans first learned to differentiate between toxic and curative plants. Palaeontologists have discovered bunches of herb, seed and flower fossils at ancient dwelling sites, confirming the belief that plant life has long been considered necessary to support human life. While herbal remedies still conjure up images of witches' brew to some, this entertaining point of view adds little to our understanding. It is only by looking to the past, understanding how central herbal medicine has been to so many ancient cultures, that we can begin to appreciate how it exerts such a powerful influence over us to this day.

Many plant, animal and mineral remedies were part of the pharmacopoeias of ancient Egyptian, Chinese and Indian civilizations. Four hundred years before Christ, Hippocrates, the father of modern medicine, utilized the healing properties of local plant life to support the healing process in his patients. A new interest grew in preventative medicine and herbal remedies continued to be used throughout Roman times. The Persians and Arabs added new remedies of their own and the knowledge of herbal medicine eventually extended to the New World.

But the New World wasn't so new and early settlers in America received a valuable education regarding local vegetation from the natives. Such has been our faith in healing plants that, in the mid-nineteenth century, traditional healers were still giving stiff competition to orthodox physicians.

It was not until the early 1900s that the active ingredients in natural substances began to be isolated in the hope that they could eventually be synthesized in the laboratory. Even today, chemists turn to Nature for inspiration. Many familiar medicines have been copied from natural blueprints. Ergometrine was copied from ergot of rye, morphine and codeine from opium poppies, atrophine from deadly nightshade, digoxin from foxglove, aspirin from white willow bark and quinine from cinchona bark. We have copied anti-ulcer drugs from liquorice and anti-cancer drugs from periwinkle and yew, and herbal medicine continues to evolve in our culture. Today there is a great interest in plants as the basis of energy medicine. The continuing development of a vast array of flower essences which cure the body by addressing the mind and emotions is testimony to this.

Herbs can be used as medicines in their own right or to complement conventional care. There are herbs to treat specific conditions, to ease pain and inflammation, relax or stimulate organs, fight bacteria and boost the immune system. Through the centuries, women have traditionally been the possessors of herbal knowledge, some were even accused of being witches and were burned at the stake because of the herbal wisdom they possessed. Women have used herbs to treat infertility and induce abortion in unwanted pregnancies. They have been used to avert miscarriage, ease the discomforts of pregnancy, strengthen contractions in labour and increase a mother's milk supply.

Herbal preparations can be taken internally or applied externally as ointments, creams and essential oils. They can be very powerful and should be taken with the same caution and respect you would take with any medication. Whether you are self-prescribing or going to a qualified herbalist, you should be prepared to ask questions: What is the herb? Is it from an organic source? What effect is it expected to have? What are the potential side-effects?

TAKING HERBAL REMEDIES

Herbal remedies can be prepared in a variety of different ways and taken internally or applied externally (*see* chart on pages 184–7). For internal use, the most common preparation is the *infusion* in which fresh or dried leaves, flowers and stems are steeped in boiling water to make a 'tea'. Harder parts of the plant, such as bark, roots, nuts and seeds will need to be boiled in a saucepan to release their therapeutic properties. This process is known as *decoction*.

Many herbal preparations also come in *tablets* and *capsules* made from the dried herb. They are also available as *tinctures*, made by steeping the raw herb in water, vinegar or alcohol. Tinctures are concentrated remedies, so you will only need to use very little each day. The usual way to take a tincture is to put a few drops in a glass of water and drink it. How much and how often you do so will vary according to the instructions on the bottle or those of your practitioner. However, some herbalists prefer tinctures to infusions and decoctions, since the dose can be more easily controlled. A tincture can also be easily absorbed, even in a body system which is very run down.

Herbs can also be used externally. You can make a herbal bath by tying fresh herbs in a muslin bag and steeping them in your bath water or by making a strong infusion or decoction and adding this to your bath. They can also be applied locally in creams and ointments, or by soaking a wash cloth in a herbal brew and using it as either a hot or cold compress. Similarly, herbal poultices – pastes made from herbal mixtures – can be applied to specific areas of the body.

Herbs in Pregnancy

Herbal remedies have similar actions on the body as conventional medicines, so should be approached with care by pregnant women. Although most of the herbs mentioned in this chapter, such as black cohosh, blue cohosh, raspberry leaf tea, squaw vine and black haw bark, have a long folk history and a wide use among midwife-herbalists, very little medical literature exists. Occasional research does surface, however, on adverse reactions to herbs. Women wishing to use herbal preparations as anything other than a mild general tonic during pregnancy and labour would be well-advised to seek the advice of a herbalist who is experienced in working with pregnancy and birth, and who can assure them of the safety of any preparations they intend to use.

Nevertheless there are demonstrated benefits of some herbal preparations. For instance, a paste made from fresh ginger, and applied before retiring to the zhiyin point on the little toe (*see* Acupuncture, page 137) has been shown to help turn breech babies into the more favourable cephalic position. In one Chinese study, more than 40 per cent of those who used the remedy experienced a spontaneous correction of the baby's position after a single treatment. After repeated treatments, 77 per cent of the babies had turned. Ginger can also be used freely to help relieve nausea during pregnancy.

Raspberry leaf tea has long been a staple of the pregnant woman's herbal medicine chest. Its main action is as a uterine tonic, but it is also rich in iron and can be useful in cases of anaemia. Although its action is considered to be entirely favourable, recent debates over the wild versus the cultivated varieties of raspberry leaf tea are a good illustration of why we should not simply regard herbs as 'natural' and therefore 'good'.

The wild variety, *Rubus strigosus*, is the herb women have been taking for centuries and upon which folk recommendations for its use in pregnancy are based. But some midwives report that the cultivated variety, *R. idaeus*, has led to miscarriage.

Raspberry leaf tea is widely available in health food shops and for most women it is unlikely to cause problems. But *R. ideaus* has received some modern scientific attention and has been found to contain caffeic acid, a substance which, in high enough doses, can suppress certain hormones necessary to maintain pregnancy. It is unlikely that an infusion of the herb would have the same effect. However, it may explain why some women experience light spotting after drinking an infusion of the herb early in pregnancy.

Because of this, women who are prone to miscarriage may wish to exercise caution with the herb until at least the 16th week of pregnancy. Women who are not prone to miscarriage can probably drink either variety through pregnancy with no ill-effects, although some practitioners still recommend limiting the intake of raspberry leaf tea to the later stages of pregnancy. Finally, a number of effective herbal remedies exist to relieve uncomfortable symptoms of pregnancy such as headache, cystitis, insomnia and heartburn. Use the chart on pages 184–7 to guide you in your choices.

EVERYDAY MEDICINE

Many herbs can be eaten as part of your daily diet. The restorative properties of oats, barley, horseradish, mustard, garlic, onion, alfalfa sprouts, seaweeds, celery, asparagus, chicory, endive, potato, carrot, artichoke, walnuts, pumpkin seeds, almonds, sesame seeds, watercress, fresh dandelion leaves, young nettles, parsley, dill, chickweed and coriander can be used – even by the most reluctant woman – as daily herbal tonics. If you are new to the idea of herbal medicine, you might want to begin your exploration of herbs by combining some of these familiar ingredients into a health-promoting and delicious daily herb salad.

HERBS IN LABOUR

The main use of herbs in labour has been to stimulate contractions. The folk tradition recommends herbs such as black cohosh, blue cohosh and squaw vine to help support the mother through the process of labour. It can be difficult, however, to know how the body will respond to herbal remedies during labour. Not all practitioners recommend the use of beneficial herbs such as black and blue cohosh because of the possibility of overstimulating the uterus. If you are unsure, remember that you can take these remedies in homeopathic form and they will be just as beneficial. What is more, you can be confident of getting a controlled dose – something which you cannot get with a simple infusion. The homeopathic remedy *Caulophyllum* is made from blue cohosh and, unlike the raw herb, has been extensively researched and found to be effective in labour. Another effective way of taking herbs in pregnancy is as a tincture. Because they are concentrated, you will not need to take much and you will be ensuring more of a standardized dose.

Nausea can often be a problem in labour and many mothers do not feel like eating or drinking during labour, though this is a vital part of maintaining even energy. Keeping a good supply of fresh ginger tea, sweetened with a little honey and lemon, can help ward off low blood sugar as well as feelings of nausea which often accompany the second, pushing stage. Ginger is also good for dealing with headaches and fatigue (though observe the cautions on page 177).

A warm-to-hot herbal compress is also a good way to help support the perineum during labour and prevent tearing. To make this, soak a wash cloth in a herbal infusion or decoction (lavender is a good choice) and apply between contractions.

WHAT TO EXPECT

Your herbalist will want to know as much about you as possible. Your initial consultation will consist of lengthy history-taking and talking about those health concerns which you feel are most important. Subsequent consultations will probably not last more than half an hour, unless your herbalist also combines other disciplines such as massage or acupuncture, into his or her practice.

Because they are so powerful, many practitioners would exercise caution in prescribing herbs during pregnancy. Before making a recommendation, any practitioner should take into account the woman's general state of health, her lifestyle, her character, the quality of support she has around her and her domestic and working environments. As pregnancy is a time of growth and nourishment, only herbs which support this process should be used.

Good choices include camomile, lime blossom, red clover, lemon balm, rose hips, cleavers, raspberry leaves, St John's wort, nasturtium, calendula, borage flowers, thyme, basil, peppermint, ginger, orange blossom and skullcap. Thoughtful use of such herbs can maintain good health and, although most health problems are self-limiting, gentle herbals can keep acute conditions from developing into chronic debilitating illnesses. You should feel free to discuss your practitioner's choice of herbs and know what to expect from each.

To find out more about herbalists in your area, contact the National Institute of Medical Herbalists or the International Register of Consultant Herbalists and Homeopaths (*see* page 302).

From a 'Master Herbalist'?

When buying commercially made herbal products, try to avoid those which are mega-blends of dozens of herbs. Pregnancy is probably not the best time to be taking large combinations of herbal remedies. Indeed, it may not be advisable at any time. Often such products are advertised as being designed by 'master' herbalists, but the claim rarely stands up to scrutiny.

A really good herbalist will choose no more than a handful of appropriate herbs in any blend. The 'everything but the kitchen sink' approach is more likely to be adopted by a master salesman or marketing executive than a master herbalist. What is more, should you have a bad reaction to a product containing multiple herbs, it will be almost impossible to say which herb or herbs caused the reaction. As far as possible keep your choices simple and you can't go wrong.

Take Care

There are a surprising number of herbs which should be avoided during the first trimester of pregnancy and, if possible, throughout the whole pregnancy. Some of the herbs which follow, such as squaw vine, blue and black cohosh may be prescribed by a qualified herbalist towards the end of pregnancy (and for a short time) to initiate an overdue labour or if there is a risk of your baby being post-mature. However, try to avoid the temptation to take such remedies on a just-in-case basis. Have some faith that your body will do its job.

Exercise caution with:

Common name	Latin name
Angelica	*Angelica archangelica*
Arbor vitae	*Thuja occidentalis*
Autumn crocus	*Colchicum autumnale*
Barberry	*Berberis vulgaris*
Beth root	*Trillium erectum*
Black cohosh*	*Cimicifuga racemose*
Blue cohosh*	*Caulophyllum thalictroides*
Broom	*Sarothamnus scoparius*
Celery seed**	*Apium graveolens*
Cotton root bark	*Gossypium hebaceum*
Fennel**	*Foeniculum vulgare*
Feverfew	*Tanacetum parthenium*
Goldenseal*	*Hydrastis canadensis*
Greater celandine	*Chelidonium majus*
Juniper	*Juniperus communis*
Lovage	*Levisticum officinale*
Meadow saffron	*Crocus sativus*
Mistletoe	*Viscum album*
Motherwort	*Leonorus cardiaca*
Mugwort	*Artemesia vulgaris*
Nutmeg**	*Myristica officinalis*
Oregano (aka Wild Marjoram)**	*Origanum vulgare*
Pennnyroyal*	*Mentha pulegium*
Peruvian bark	*Cinchona officinalis*
Poke root	*Phytolacca decandra*

Rosemary**	*Rosemarinus officinalis*
Rue	*Ruta graveolens*
Sage**	*Salvia officinalis*
Sassafrass	*Sassafrass officinalis*
Squaw vine*	*Mitchella repens*
Tansy	*Tanacetum vulgare*
Thyme**	*Thymus vulgaris*
Vervain	*Verbena officinalis*
Wormwood	*Artemesia absinthum*

These herbs can be used in labour and may be effective in cases of threatened miscarriage. Consult your practitioner.

*** These common culinary herbs are generally safe, especially when used in culinary quantities. However, if you are prone to miscarriage you may wish to avoid them.*

Perhaps the most famous case report of an adverse reaction to herbs is what's come to be known in herbal lore as 'the hairy baby story', where a woman taking large amounts of Siberian ginseng to relieve depression during pregnancy gave birth to a highly androgynous baby, covered with thick black hair, and with swollen testes and swollen red nipples. Although the baby eventually recovered, this tale highlights the folly of gulping down massive doses of anything while pregnant.

Care should be taken with a few other common herbal remedies. Avoid herbal laxatives such as aloe, cascara and senna, since these can stimulate contractions. St John's wort, used to treat depression during pregnancy, has no reported toxic effects but should still be used with caution due to the possibility that it can stimulate uterine contractions.

Ginger can be very helpful in relieving exhaustion during labour. However, since it can also increase circulation to all parts, including the womb, it may be best to avoid it in the later stages of labour, when it may increase the risk of post partum haemorrhage.

TRY IT YOURSELF

When buying herbal teas and remedies for yourself, be selective. The widely available herbal teas, such as those in most supermarkets, may not have any caffeine, but they often have very little therapeutic value and contain flavourings which may be derived from chemical sources. In a specialist health food shop, you are likely to find a wider range of herbal teas with no additives (some are even organic) and which will have mild therapeutic effects.

The chart on pages 184–7 provides a list of some of the most helpful herbs to use in pregnancy and labour. You may wish to use it as a guideline for putting together a basic herbal pregnancy and labour kit. The most useful herbals for each condition are highlighted in italics to make selection easier for beginners. Self-prescription is a safe option, but remember that no remedy should be taken long-term unless under the guidance of a qualified herbalist.

FLOWER ESSENCES

It is said that there are no diseases, only sick people. This could best describe the philosophy of those who practise energy medicine, and in particular those who use flower essences.

Ancient philosophers maintained that life, or matter, was composed of energy and that all body processes were simply patterns of energy. The presence of health or sickness was ultimately directed by subtle movements and changes in those patterns. Modern medicine aims for stasis – a suppression of 'undesirable' symptoms – whereas to ancient practitioners movement was natural, even desirable, because where there is movement there is life.

The various forms of energy medicine – homeopathy, acupuncture, kinesiology, healing and meditation – see the life force as something which sustains and organizes the physical body. The aim is to transform energy patterns directly, using various techniques to stimulate the body in the direction of greater balance and the removal of disease. In contrast, conventional medicine treats only the results of these shifts in energy, and conventional doctors dispute the existence of a life force because it is difficult to measure. If it can't be measured, doctors argue, how can you be sure that it works?

Dr Edward Bach (pronounced *batch*), an English bacteriologist and homeopath, is generally credited with the discovery of the healing properties of potentized plant essences. Using his grounding in both conventional science and intuitive diagnosis, he began to develop his own individual theories on the way that personality types – first 12, then 19 and finally 38 different types, corresponding to the 38 remedies in today's Bach repertory – influenced disease and how this effect could be mediated by the use of certain plant essences. Unfortunately, Bach kept none of his research papers, lectured infrequently and preferred to diagnose intuitively, so his method of observing plants and ascribing various energies to them remains shrouded in mystery. But it is a mystery which suits the esoteric healers, who rely heavily on his and other flower remedies, since it has left the field wide open for a large diversity of practitioners to use and develop flower essences in their own ways, an intuitive and creative practice which sometimes creates more confusion than health.

Today, in addition to the 38 classic remedies of Dr Bach, there are 72 Australian Bush Essences, 102 Californian Essences, the Alaskan Flower Essences, the Findhorn Flower Essences from Scotland, the Bailey Flower Essences from Yorkshire, the Himalayan Essences and more general combination essences from any number of media-friendly healers. On the fringe there are also environmental, colour and light essences, gem and crystal essences and chakra essences to be found almost everywhere in the world.

It is hard to imagine that any of these could be very different from each other, and the sheer number of flower essences being developed and promoted is simply overwhelming. Nevertheless, their manufacturers claim subtle differences in their approach. Bach and the Australian essences, for example, are both very much grounded in the day-to-day, physical world, although the Australian essences address more specific concerns, such as sexuality, communication, spirituality and learning, rather than personality type. The Californian Essences work on a more esoteric level, and the Himalayan and Alaskan essences, rather like their places of origin, can only be described as targeting the more remote parts of the human psyche.

Flower essences can be used on their own or in a complementary way with orthodox medicine. They work gently with emotions and the psyche, enabling a person to deal with any conflicts or problems at a pace which suits them.

MAKING YOUR OWN ESSENCES

While walking through the woods near his Oxfordshire home, Dr Bach gathered dewdrops from flowers, plants and trees. He used these to make remedies which he tested on himself. He began to notice that dewdrops exposed to sunlight were more potent than those which were not.

This knowledge evolved into what is known as the 'sunlight method'. You can use this method to make your own simple flower essences. Here's what to do:

• Pick your flowers by hand, preferably in the early morning hours at the peak of their bloom.
• Place the flowers in a glass container containing spring water or purified water. The flowers should cover the surface of the water.

• Leave the container in direct sunlight for around three hours or until the flowers begin to wilt.
• Remove the flowers with a clean utensil, or, if you prefer the rustic approach, a twig.
• Pour the remaining liquid into an amber dropper bottle half-filled with brandy or glycerine (which is used as a preservative).
• Shake vigorously and label.

The resulting liquid, called a 'mother tincture', will keep for many years if properly stored (in a dark bottle in cool conditions). To make a stock remedy from your mother tincture place two drops of mother tincture into a 1fl oz (30ml) dropper bottle containing a teaspoon of brandy and then fill with spring water. This remedy can then be taken in water or on the tongue.

Use your common sense. A great deal of literature exists to assist you in choosing only those flowers which are known to be non-poisonous and non-addictive. Avoid those which grow by busy roadsides and which have been treated with pesticides. To make sure you get the best and most appropriate flowers, consider turning a patch of your own garden into a medicinal flower garden.

The various manufacturers also claim considerable differences in the uses of essences made from the same species of plant. This begs a perfectly fair question: why, for instance, should the properties of a poppy from Europe be so fundamentally different from one grown in California?

The answer, according to devotees, would be that different parts of the world radiate different energy patterns. The mineral content of different soils, a plant's ability to thrive, the time it is harvested and even the people involved in the harvesting, manufacture and prescription of the remedy all have a profound effect on its efficacy. Considering how potentially complex the argument can get, it is easy to see why Dr Bach advised patients and practitioners alike to close off their minds to such explanations completely! It is also easy to see why many practitioners adhere to the tried-and-tested, well-catalogued (and relatively few) remedies of Dr Bach.

Many practitioners find that chronic illnesses – everything from hayfever and asthma to ME and lupus – which do not respond to conventional treatment, respond favourably to flower remedies. Certainly there are no known adverse interactions with conventional medicine, making flower essences a good choice to complement conventional regimes.

TAKING FLOWER REMEDIES

So many women swear by flower remedies, no matter how they work, that they must be considered a valid choice in any natural medicine chest. Because they come in small bottles and can be placed directly on the tongue or sipped from a glass of water, flower remedies are among the most portable medicines a woman can use. Since they work very gently and have no known side-effects, it's worth experimenting to find a remedy that is right for you.

Most alternative practitioners will recommend that you choose your remedy intuitively according to your needs. Many will recommend flower remedies either on their own or in conjunction with any other remedy they may prescribe.

To learn more about flower essences, contact Bach Flower Remedies or the Flower Essence Fellowship (*see* page 302).

FLOWER REMEDIES FOR PREGNANCY AND BIRTH

A full exploration of flower remedies is beyond the scope of this book, but the following remedies are particularly suitable for pregnancy and labour:

Rescue Remedy is the original combination remedy invented by Bach. It contains Rock Rose, Clematis, Impatiens, Cherry Plum and Star of Bethlehem. There are many imitators on the market which claim to do much the same thing. However, Rescue Remedy is the best known and can be used whenever you feel fearful, anxious, exhausted or ill. Labouring women find Rescue Remedy particularly effective. However, it is appropriate for any emergency application.

Olive is the classic remedy for total physical exhaustion. Useful for those who have lost their sense of optimism and the will to struggle on.

Walnut helps to manage periods of transition and integrate the change into your life.

Willow is used for those with a negative outlook, and a feeling that nothing is fair. This type of person complains about an experience instead of learning from it.

Mimulus is for paralysing fear of something, in this case childbirth.

Hornbeam can be used to alleviate lassitude, procrastination and a 'Monday morning' feeling.

Mustard is effective for gloom which descends for no apparent reason.

Gentian is helpful when you are feeling uncertain of the right path to take and can't make a decision.

Some practitioners believe that individuals should only take essences derived from flowers which are common to their own country. Nevertheless, good results can be obtained with remedies from other countries. For instance, among the Californian Essences good choices are:

Arnica for keeping your feet on the ground, helping to recover from any trauma – mental, emotional or physical. Identical to homeopathic arnica.

Pomegranate is a good choice for modern women who are having trouble reconciling the often conflicting demands of home and career, husband and child.

Alpine lily is a female remedy which relates to positive and negative attitudes toward the body and sexuality.

And from Australia...

Crowea for when you've got into the habit of worrying but you can't recall exactly why this is. This remedy is reputed to help find the answer.

Sturt Desert pea is for when you feel trapped by some past hurt and are unable to express your feelings about it. Such a situation can keep you from moving on or may also cause chronic physical illnesses.

Waratah for periods of intense changes which you find impossible to keep up with. It counters loss of faith in yourself, in humanity and in those around you. Has potential to help in labour.

Which Herbs can Help?

Symptom	Internally	Externally	In your diet	Other comments
Anaemia	Nettle, Comfrey, Yellow dock, Rosehips, Burdock, Gentian	None	Include plenty of watercress, fresh dandelion leaves, nettle tops, lambs' lettuce, parsley, chicory, seaweeds and spring onions. Try also fresh pressed beetroot juice. Kelp is a rich source of iron	Vitamin C aids the absorption of iron so boost your intake with, preferably, a glass of citrus juice, or supplements, at mealtimes
Backache	Nettles or cleavers may sometimes be indicated to ease back pain around the kidneys. Comfrey may help strengthen muscles	Try a herbal bath with ginger, lavender, rosemary or mustard	Try including foods rich in vitamins C and B complex – wheatgrass juice is very suitable	External remedies listed here are also appropriate for a backache during labour
Candida	Echinacea, cleavers and camomile are immune system restoratives. Use any of the above in combination with marigold, wild indigo, golden rod, ground ivy and plantain to strengthen mucous memranes	Try a compress made with marigold, camomile, American cranesbill, beth root, echinacea, cleavers, wild indigo or use any of these in your bath. Tea tree in the bath may also help	Lots of garlic and olive oil both of which discourage the growth of fungi. Also include raw kale, turnip, cabbage, which inhibit fungal growth	You can pass candida on to your child during birth, so deal with it now. No sugar, no spices, loose cotton underwear and plenty of live plain yoghurt
Constipation	Dandelion root, fennel, beetroot fibre, pysllium husk	None	Include lots of water-soluble seeds, such as linseed and flax, in salads on top of yoghurts and cereals, etc.	Stay away from processed and 'junk' foods and drink plenty of water
Cramp	Cramp bark, nettle, hawthorn leaves, flower and berries, meadowsweet	None	Potato, carrot, celery, greens, onions and garlic are rich in potassium to help alleviate cramp. Make a soup using each of these	Cramp can sometimes indicate inadequate salt intake

Condition	Herbs			
Cystitis	*Marshmallow*, horsetail, couchgrass, *cornsilk*, meadowsweet, *nettle*, *marigold*, liquorice root. If there is fever: *uva ursi*, *yarrow*, plantain or agrimony	None	Unsweetened cranberry juice can halt the progress of the infection. You can usually find this at health food shops only. Make your own barley water by cooking barley with plenty of water, strain off mix with a little lemon juice and sip throughout the day	Begin treatment at the first sign of discomfort to avoid the condition becoming chronic or spreading to other parts of the urinary system. Cystitis is often linked to Candida so follow similar dietary measures
Fluid retention	Raspberry leaf, *dandelion leaves*, *cleavers*, couchgrass, horsetail, *cornsilk*	None	Include more grapes, asparagus and apples in your diet. Dandelion leaves in a salad will also help maintain water balance	Fluid retention on its own is not dangerous so don't panic. *Never take diuretics*
Haemorrhoids	*Yellow dock*, *dandelion*, *nettle* and oat straw will strengthen your system	Cool compresses made with tinctures of *witch hazel*, plantain, *marshmallow root*, *oak bark*. Comfrey, mullein, hawthorn berry are comforting. Proprietary *pilewort* ointment can be purchased in most health food stores	Incude plenty of garlic, onion, parsley, dandelion root, lime blossom and ginger	A high fibre diet will prevent straining. You can buy herbal ointments and creams from most health food shops
Headache	To relieve stress: *skullcap*, lemon balm, *passion flower*, *lime flowers*, camomile. For migraine: *feverfew*	Try a steam inhalation of *peppermint* or lavender. Alternatively use a cool compress with rosemary and lavender	Vascular symptoms can be lessened with a diet rich in garlic and onions	Headaches are symptoms, not diseases. Most are caused by stress (physical and emotional). Removing the stress usually removes the headache
Heartburn	*Meadowsweet*, camomile, *peppermint*, *lemon verbena*, marshmallow, liquorice. Slippery elm powder can be taken as a lozenge or mixed into a drink	None	When cooking, try to include more fennel, anise, caraway and dill	Meals should be little and often rather than three main meals a day. Chew food thoroughly and avoid spicy or greasy foods
Hypertension	*Hawthorn berry*, skullcap, *passion flower*, hops	None	Garlic, onion and parsley can help to keep blood moving smoothly through the veins. Cucumber can also help to lower blood pressure	Hypertension requires a variety of approaches so consider stress-reducing techniques such as yoga and meditation

Which Herbs can Help?

IN PREGNANCY continued

Symptom	Internally	Externally	In your diet	Other comments
Insomnia	Mild sedatives: *skullcap, oat camomile,* lavender, raspberry leaf, *lime tree flower, passion flower.* Stronger sedatives: *valerian,* hops	Buy or make a herbal sleep pillow. To make one pillow stuff a small pillowcase (you can sew one yourself) with lavender, camomile, lime flowers and hops. Sew up the end and place this under your head as you sleep. The weight of your head will crush the herbs and release soothing scent	None	Always begin by trying mild sedatives first. These can be drunk as tea or taken as tincture throughout the day and won't make you spaced out. Stronger sedatives should only be taken at night. Do not take valerian in the first trimester
Miscarriage	Before 14 weeks: decoctions of *cramp bark or black haw bark* can relax uterine muscle. After 14 weeks: chasteberry or *false unicorn root* tincture normalize hormone function. Any time: *raspberry leaf* is a general uterine tonic; to soothe anxiety *skullcap, lime blossom* and lemon balm. To complete a miscarriage: *black cohosh, blue cohosh*	None	Diet should include iron-rich foods (see Anaemia) and plenty of garlic to ward off infection	Always consult your practitioner if you suspect miscarriage
Nausea	*Ginger,* Roman camomile, dandelion, *peppermint.* With vomiting: *Black horehound* mixed with spearmint to mask the taste.	None	Use ginger liberally in your cooking	Excessive vomiting, called hyperemesis, can drain your body of essential nutrients. Consult your practitioner if you are experiencing this. The remedies listed here are also useful in labour

Which Herbs can Help?

Contractions – encouraging, strengthening	Traditionally, *squaw vine* aids labour. Stronger herbs such as *blue cohosh* and *goldenseal* should be used carefully, perhaps under the guidance of a qualified practitioner. *Raspberry leaf* helps maintain uterine tone	None	Iron-rich foods will help the uterine muscle work more efficiently (see Anaemia above)	Muscles need glucose to work. Keep blood sugar levels high by eating small light snacks throughout labour – see pages 104–105 for appropriate foods
Pain	General: tincture of *motherwort* or *skullcap* can help relieve any anxiety and tension. Cramp: *crampbark* and St John's wort can help relieve cramping pain. Afterpains: Catnip tincture	None	None	Maintaining an upright position will assist your contractions. When the uterus does not have to work so hard, pain is more manageable
Perineal support	None	In labour: a very hot compress soaked in an infusion of *lavender* or camomile. Use in between second stage contractions. Swollen, bruised or torn: warm decoction of *oak bark*, comfrey bark, marigold and lavender flowers. Use a compress or in a shallow basin for bathing the perineal area. Alternatively, bathe the wound in a solution of calendula tincture and water. *Witch hazel* eases bruising	Zinc-rich food, herbs and roots such as ginger, parsley, potatoes, garlic, turnips, carrots, rye, oats and buckwheat will all aid skin healing	Bed rest is important to help aid perineal healing. Even women who do not tear need time to recover. For bruising, try soaking sanitary pads in the herbal solution of your choice and freezing them. Wearing these is more comfortable than the pack of frozen peas usually recommended
Placenta (expelling)	*Angelica*, *ground ivy*, goldenseal, raspberry leaf, *nettle*	None	None	Don't panic if your placenta doesn't immediately follow the baby. It can take up to an hour to complete this third stage of labour. Putting your baby to the breast soon after birth will help
Recovery	*Nettle*, *motherwort*, lemon balm, hawthorn berry, leaf and flower, fennel	Compress (hot or cold) with *lavender* can help relieve perineal pain	Make sure you are eating iron-rich foods (see Anaemia) and zinc-rich foods (see Perineal support)	Rest is essential after even the most straightforward birth. It gives body and mind a chance to adjust

CHAPTER 13

HOMEOPATHY

WHAT IT'S BEST FOR

HAEMORRHOIDS

CARPAL TUNNEL SYNDROME

NAUSEA/VOMITING

ANXIETY

DEPRESSION

INDUCE/ACCELERATE LABOUR

RESPIRATORY PROBLEMS

CONSTIPATION

CYSTITIS

CRAMP

FEAR

HEADACHE

HEARTBURN

TURNING A BREECH

INSOMNIA

COLDS AND FLU

☑ **Some conditions require a professional therapist**
☑ **Some conditions are suitable for simple self-treatment**

Pregnancy is a good time to discover homeopathy ...

For many women their first experimentation with homeopathic medicines occurs when they are pregnant. Some are attracted by the fact that homeopathy offers a safe and effective way to deal with minor complaints, others are investigating a more natural approach to potential difficulties in labour. Either way, the non-toxic, widely available remedies used in homeopathy make an attractive choice.

In homeopathy infinitesimal doses of medicines derived from a variety of plant, mineral, chemical and even animal sources are used. These minute doses are capable of producing change and enhancing the body's own capacity for both physical and emotional healing. Homeopathy is based on the idea that like can cure like, or the 'law of similars'. This idea was well known to the ancient Greeks but was only resurrected in Western society in the eighteenth century when a German physician, Samuel Hahnemann, began looking for a more humane way to treat his patients.

During his years as a physician, Hahnemann became increasingly distressed by the often barbaric cures of his day which included bleeding, purging and the use of leeches. Eventually he chose to leave the medical profession altogether, supporting his family by translating medical, scientific and botanical texts. While engaged in this work he uncovered the ancient law of similars. His first application of this principle was to test the effect of chinchona bark which was, at the time, a common treatment for malaria. During his research, he noted that in healthy individuals the bark could produce malaria-like symptoms, but when tiny doses of homeopathic chinchona were administered to malaria patients, their symptoms abated.

Hahnemann's approach was, and still is, a complete contrast to conventional medicine, which traditionally treats a patient's symptoms with medicines which have the opposite effect. So, for example, a person suffering from insomnia would be given something to induce an artificial sleep. In homeopathy, this same person would be given a minute dose of something such as coffea (derived from unroasted coffee), which would normally act as a stimulant and which in a healthy adult would produce sleeplessness.

Having rediscovered the law of similars, Hahnemann spent the rest of his life developing and cataloguing the relationship between diseases and symptoms and the toxic effects of natural medically active substances. Today, more than 2,000 substances, describing symptom patterns of the most common conditions such as allergy, cold, flu and bruises, have been catalogued. Professional homeopaths use relatively few of these in their day-to-day practice and you certainly do not need to be an expert in all

2,000 to learn to diagnose and prescribe safely and effectively for yourself.

Homeopathy has been the subject of a great deal of medical scrutiny over the last few years. For instance, in 1997 when the respected medical journal *The Lancet* conducted a thorough review of all the properly conducted clinical trials into homeopathy published between 1943 and 1995, it concluded that 77 per cent of these studies yielded a positive result. In addition, while some conventional practitioners pooh-pooh the effectiveness of homeopathy as a mere 'placebo effect', in this review homeopathy was ten times more effective than placebos.

Unlike conventional drugs, homeopathic remedies do not cause side-effects and you cannot become addicted to them. Although many people report a swift and profound relief from their symptoms with homeopathy, most studies show that homeopathy tends to work slowly, but produces long-lasting results.

Homeopathic remedies are available in a bafflingly wide range of doses from specialist suppliers. However, the remedies which you can buy in most health food shops are commonly sold in two strengths, 6C and 30C (though occasionally the C is omitted on the label). This is a centesimal dose, meaning that the remedy has been diluted 1 part remedy to 99 parts water and alcohol.

In a 6C remedy, for example, the remedy will have been diluted and shaken vigorously to release its energy. One part of this newly diluted solution will then be mixed with 99 parts water and alcohol, and the process can be repeated any number of times to achieve the desired potency. (For example, in a 6C remedy this process will have taken place six times.) Less is more in homeopathy and although the 30C remedy has been diluted more times it is considered more potent.

It is important if you are self-diagnosing and buying homeopathic remedies over the counter not to use them as you would a conventional remedy. Often a single dose is all that is required. This is something which can be very difficult to take on board if you have spent years taking medicine on a three- or four-times-daily schedule. If you are uncertain about how to take a remedy and the remedy's label is unclear, it is best to consult a qualified therapist for advice.

If you or your homeopath select the wrong remedy it simply won't work and you will not suffer any unpleasant side-effects. If the right remedy has been chosen, some change may take place within a relatively short time. It is important to remember that once a change does occur you should stop taking the remedy (don't be tempted even to take another dose 'for luck'); your body will take over the process from then on.

How does it work?

Doctors and scientists have developed many different theories in order to explain how such infinitesimal doses of a pharmacologically active substance can produce such profound results. One of the more intriguing is the 'memory of water' theory. Chemists believe that when the active ingredient is mixed in the water/alcohol base and shaken vigorously it makes an imprint on the water. Even though none of the active ingredient remains after this process, the water retains information about the active ingredient in this imprint even after millions of dilutions. What is more, repeated dilutions, known as potentizations, make the imprint stronger, not weaker, which is why higher dilutions are considered stronger medicine.

HOMEOPATHY IN PREGNANCY

The large dilutions used in homeopathy are well suited to conditions in pregnancy since they have been show to be free from adverse side-effects, even if the wrong remedy is selected. When the right remedy is selected, it can produce health benefits for the woman which may remain long after she has given birth.

Although homeopathic remedies can be selected to treat specific conditions such as heartburn, insomnia, constipation and cramp, some of the best long-term treatments involve treating the pregnant woman constitutionally. What this means is that instead of targeting individual symptoms, the homeopath will prescribe a remedy which matches the woman's personality, emotions and lifestyle. When each of these elements is in harmony, the woman will generally find that nagging physical complaints tend to fade away.

For women who are interested in breaking family health patterns homeopathy can be extremely useful. Many practitioners report success in healing inherited conditions such as varicosities and illnesses such as asthma and eczema.

Although it is not always thought of as a first line of treatment, homeopathy is also an effective way of breaking emotional patterns. Anxiety, depression, fear, lack of confidence and apathy can all be treated with properly selected remedies.

HOMEOPATHY IN LABOUR

Among the most successful uses of homeopathy are in stimulating contractions in labour and easing labour pains. For this purpose the remedy *Caulophyllum* has received the most attention for its ability to strengthen contractions and assist dilation. *Caulophyllum* has been the subject of several homeopathic studies and all the available literature suggests that its use can help to shorten the duration of labour, in some cases by as much as 90 minutes.

If you have experienced a previous labour where your contractions were not terribly efficient or powerful, your practitioner may recommend that you begin by taking *Caulophyllum*, or another suitable remedy such as *Secale*, or *Pulsatilla* (*see* table, pages 199–205) before term. There is some evidence, both scientific and anecdotal, that doing this from around your 38th week of pregnancy may prevent potential problems recurring in labour.

Even if you do not wish to or need to use homeopathic remedies to help your labour, you may wish to keep some for use after birth. The single most important of these will be *Arnica,* which can ease painful breasts and help assist the healing of any bruises or tears. Even women with no perineal tears or episiotomy cuts may experience pain in this area and *Arnica* is the remedy of choice. If you feel shocked after the birth of your child the remedy *Aconite* is indicated. Most practitioners would recommend that both *Arnica* and *Aconite* should be included in every woman's basic pregnancy and birth kit.

WHAT TO EXPECT

Your homeopath will want to take a full medical history from you and this will take up most of your first session together. Once the history-taking is completed, your practitioner will study your pattern of symptoms and choose a remedy which is best for you. A traditional homeopath will generally prescribe a single remedy which will treat you constitutionally. You may be given this in a single, very high dose or in a lower potency taken over a period of days.

Other homeopaths, believing that there are no 'true' types, prefer to address symptom patterns and may prescribe combination remedies. There is disagreement among practitioners about which method is 'officially' best and which reflects true homeopathic practice. In self-prescribing you can treat constitutionally or in a symptom-oriented way, since over-the-counter remedies are available both singly and in combination form. A great deal of literature exists to help self-prescribers identify major symptom patterns and personality types and assist you in your choices.

Professional homeopaths generally distinguish between acute symptoms, which they see as representing self-protective efforts by the body and/or psyche to deal with recent stress or infection, and chronic symptoms, recurrent, unsuccessful efforts by the body to re-establish health. Chronic symptoms may persist if you are weakened by stress, lifestyle or environmental factors or because of some inherited weakness. Sometimes what appears to be an acute condition is really the manifestation of an underlying chronic condition. This is just one example of a case where a 'constitutional remedy', which matches the *totality* of the symptoms, may be particularly appropriate.

To Western women, who are used to being prescribed single pills for single problems, this may seem a strange way of doing things. The reason why this type of prescribing is important, however, becomes apparent when looking at conditions such as morning sickness. Nausea in pregnancy can have many causes; it can have a physical cause such as hormonal fluctuations, food sensitivity or environmental allergens. But it can also be triggered by emotional factors such as stress, fear of being pregnant, anxiety and isolation.

A homeopath, through taking a careful history and talking through a woman's feelings about being pregnant, will be better able to help her understand more about the cause of her nausea and choose an appropriate remedy. In some cases, if the woman is very ill and experiencing unremitting nausea, indigestion, diarrhoea and vomiting, the homeopath may work first with the acute symptoms and then, when things have settled down, prescribe a different remedy to deal with the underlying cause.

In most cases, once a remedy is selected you will not need to see your practitioner again too soon. It will be apparent if the right remedy has been selected, since you will begin to note a progressive improvement in your condition and your practitioner may only need to see you again in two weeks' or a month's time to check your progress. Nevertheless, during pregnancy, some women make a monthly appointment with their homeopath just to maintain links and to help deal with any new symptoms which crop up as pregnancy progresses.

To contact a homeopath in your local area, get in touch with the British Homeopathic Association or the Society of Homeopaths (*see* pages 303–5).

Take Care

There are very few cautions with homeopathy. Most homeopaths do not recommend taking daily doses of any remedy for extended periods of time. Generally speaking, if there has not been some form of improvement within a week or so, you may want to consider another remedy. There is absolutely no evidence that homeopathic remedies can cause any adverse effects in either a mother or her unborn child. However, women with a history of miscarriage should avoid taking the remedies *Apis, Silicea* or *Thuja,* as these may increase their risk of another miscarriage.

Studies relating to pregnancy and birth have generally focused on ways to hasten labour and many have shown good results with carefully selected remedies. However, it's important to read between the lines. Faster labours are not always 'best' labours. Any remedy which has the potential to strengthen contractions also, theoretically, has the power to produce, in some women, the problems associated with any artificially strengthened contractions. These may include more fetal distress and more cervical and perineal tears. Never assume, or allow anyone else to assume, that your body isn't going to work properly. Just-in-case medicine is no more appropriate in alternative medicine than it is in conventional medicine.

The Tissue Salts

The remedies known as tissue salts exist on the border between homeopathic and nutritional medicine. Although they are diluted in the same way they are not diluted to the same degree. Instead they come in a decimal potency (usually 6X), as opposed to the centesimal, or C, potencies common to other homeopathic remedies. This means that they have been diluted six times, one part remedy to ten parts water and alcohol. At this level of dilution there is even a theoretical possibility that some of the original material remains.

Your body tissues are made up, in part, of various inorganic minerals also known as biochemical cell salts. There are 12 tissue salts in all, each of them playing a role in maintaining the health of our bodies. During pregnancy the balance of tissue salts in the body changes according to the demands of your growing baby. Occasionally this can result in deficiency which can show itself as uncomfortable physical symptoms such as cramp or constipation.

Tissue salts can be purchased as single remedies or in combination, in most chemists and health food shops. Five of the twelve are particularly relevant during pregnancy. These are:

• **Natrum mur (chloride of soda)** Regulates the body's water balance and carries moisture to the cells. Imbalance may result in salt cravings, hay fever, and watery discharges from the eyes and nose. This remedy may also prevent heartburn, swollen ankles and dry skin.

• **Ferum phos (phosphate of iron)** A constituent of the blood and other body tissues. Imbalance may cause diarrhoea, constipation and even spontaneous nose bleeds. This remedy is occasionally helpful in cases of anaemia.

• **Mag phos (phosphate of magnesia)** A component of the teeth, bones, brain, blood, nerves and muscle cells. Deficiency can cause cramp, neuralgia and shooting pains.

• **Calc fluor (fluoride of lime)** Found in all your body's connective tissues. Imbalance can result in varicosities, muscle tendon strain and cracked, dry skin. This remedy is often recommended to prevent stretch marks.

• **Silica (silicic acid)** Exists in all connective tissue as well as in hair, skin and nails. Imbalance or deficiency can result in poor memory, thinning hair and ribbed or ingrowing nails.

Tissue salts are finely balanced in the body and you may not need to take more than one tablet daily on alternate weeks to effect change. If unsure, consult your practitioner.

USING THE CHART

The chart on pages 199–205 is a summary of some of the most effective homeopathic remedies used in pregnancy and labour. Both 6C and 30C potencies are appropriate for most of the conditions a woman will experience during pregnancy. As a general guideline, the higher 30C potency acts more quickly and deeply than the lower 6C potency, but requires a more precise selection of an appropriate remedy. If after selecting a remedy from the chart, you are unsure about which potency to use, start with the lower potency. For many conditions the right choice of remedy may be more important than its potency. Nevertheless, a useful guideline when self-prescribing is to try to match the potency to the nature of the symptoms; select a 6C potency for chronic conditions which have been slow to develop and which seem neither to improve nor get worse, and 30C for those which come on quickly and are more intense.

How frequently you take the remedy depends on the urgency of the situation. Thus, for mild morning sickness you may need only one tablet day and night and for other chronic conditions no more than three 6C tablets daily. Higher potencies should be taken less frequently. For example, in cases of anxiety, a severe backache or a headache which comes on suddenly, a single 30C potency would be appropriate. In urgent, changeable situations, such as during labour, you could conceivably take one 30C tablet every five or ten minutes for up to four to six doses, or your homeopath or midwife might prescribe a single very high potency (200C or more) tablet.

Selection of the right remedy, in the right potency, is only one part of the process, however. Taking your remedies under the right conditions and storing them properly will also ensure that your homeopathic remedies work optimally for you. Homeopathic remedies are very delicate and certain things will act as an antidote to them. Try following these guidelines to get the best out of your remedies:

• You should not touch homeopathic remedies with your bare hands. Always tip them straight into the bottle top and from there into your mouth. To make this process easier, some commercially available remedies now come in single-dose dispensers. Remedies should always be stored in a cool, dark place. Do not store them near any essential oils or electronic devices.

• You should not take a remedy less than 20 minutes before or after food. Also avoid strong, highly flavoured foods and other items such as mints (toothpaste, gum, mouthwash, etc.), cloves, garlic or onions immediately before or after taking a remedy. Products containing eucalyptus and camphor will also act as an antidote to your remedies as will cigarette smoke and caffeine. While you are taking a homeopathic remedy it may be wise to switch to a non-mint toothpaste. There are several on the market but those flavoured with fennel are a particularly good choice. It is also advisable not to wear strong perfumes while taking remedies, since these can sometimes act as an antidote.

• Homeopathic remedies may also be damaged by the electromagnetic fields generated by telephones, cell phones, headphones, computers and by machines with large motors, such as automobiles. It's probably best to avoid these for five minutes before taking a remedy and for 25 minutes afterwards.

Which Homeopathic Remedy?

FOR PREGNANCY

Condition	Symptoms	What makes it better?	What makes it worse?	Suggested remedy
Anxiety/Fear	Comes on suddenly	Open air, rest, warm sweat	Cold dry wind, getting chilled, night, fright, shock, noise, light	Aconite
	Weeping for no apparent reason	Open air, cold dry air, cold food, cool applications, gentle movement, sympathy, consolation	Heat and stuffy rooms, emotional upset, humidity, too many clothes or bedclothes	Pulsatilla
	Accompanied by nervousness, lethargy	Warmth, rest, food	Excitement, worry, mental and physical exertion, cold, early morning, eating	Kali phos (tissue salt)
Backache	Back feels weak and tired, dragging pains in middle and lower back	Open air, sitting bent over, warmth of any kind	Morning 2am–5am, cold, chill, damp, worse lying on affected side, exertion especially sexually, during and after eating, getting too hot	Kali carb
	Comes on suddenly; pain can be intense, often right-sided, can be accompanied by abdominal pain head may feel hot	Pressure, rest, warmth, light warm wraps	Jarring motion, touch, pressure, cold, light noise, lying on the painful side, heat	Belladonna
	Intense spasmodic pain, tense feeling in abdomen, feeling chilly	Sleep, nap, heat, warmth, evenings, warm shower or compress, firm pressure	Morning on waking, after meals coffee, alcohol, cold, cold dry weather, cold dry winds, spices, overwork, anger, sedentary lifestyle, loss of sleep	Nux vomica

Which Homeopathic Remedy?

FOR PREGNANCY continued

Condition	Symptoms	What makes it better?	What makes it worse?	Suggested remedy
Constipation	Dry hard stools or difficulty passing even soft stools, straining	Open air, cold washing, in the evenings, comes on alternate days, damp weather	Afternoons, sedentary lifestyle, potatoes, alternate days	Alumina
	Straining to pass a stool, irritability	Heat, warmth, sleep or a nap, evenings, bath or a shower, firm pressure	Morning on waking, after meals, coffee, alcohol, cold, cold dry weather, cold dry winds, overwork, anger, sedentary lifestyle, loss of sleep	Nux vomica
	Incomplete bowel movement with flatulence	Outside in the open air, motion, warm drinks, lying on left side	Away from home, 4pm–8pm from cold air, cold drinks, warm rooms, restrictive clothing	Lycopodium
	Stubborn constipation lasts days feels like there's a ball in the rectum	Eating, vigorous exercise, running, fast walking, dancing, elevating the legs	Cold, fasting, getting wet, rest, swimming, mental exertion, kneeling, storm brewing, morning and early evening	Sepia
Cramp	Cramping, radiating pains, in the calves, sciatica, tender feet, symptoms common to office workers and sports people	Warmth, pressure, bending double, friction, hot liquids	Right side, cold touch, at night, tight clothing	Mag phos (tissue salt)
	Pins and needles in arms and legs, soles of feet	Rest, evenings, in damp/wet weather, strong pressure	Cold, morning, dry cold weather dry cold winds	Nux vomica
	Legs feel cold and numb, cracking in joints	Cold weather, putting feet in cold water	Heat, nighttime	Ledum

	Symptoms	Better for	Worse for	Remedy
Cystitis	Frequent urge to pass urine, clingy, tearful and weepy	Open air, cold dry air, cold food, cool applications, pressure, gentle movement, sympathy, consolation	Heat and stuffy rooms, humidity too many clothes or bedclothes, fatty foods, emotional upset	Pulsatilla
	Comes on suddenly, fever, hot, dry skin, restless and irritable	Peace and quiet, warmth, sitting up in bed, darkened rooms	Cold and chill, bright lights, noise, pregnancy, jolting or jarring movement	Belladonna
	Ineffectual urge to urinate or incomplete evacuation, easily angered and irritable	After breakfast, warmth, rest	Early morning, intercourse, after surgery or hi-tech birth, anger, indignation, grief	Staphysagria
Haemorrhoids	Sore, raw, bleeding feeling as if piles will burst	n/a	Warm, moist air	Hamamemelis
	Internal (blind) piles with backache, constipation and bleeding	Heat, warm applications	Pregnancy, rest, changes of weather	Calc fluor
	Itching, burning oozing with constipation or painless diarrhoea	Warm dry weather, lying on right side	In a warm bed, standing, bathing, mid-morning, night, alcohol	Sulphur
	Distended bluish veins, burning pain after bowel movovement	Cool air, sleep, breaking wind	Evening, night, after eating fatty foods, alcohol	Carbo veg
Headache	Band-like pain especially over the eyes, dizziness and exhaustion	Bending forwards, perspiring, lying with head elevated	Stress, movement, heat, sunlight smoking hot, damp weather	Gelsemium
	Severe, throbbing pain often with constipation, sensitive scalp	Firm pressure, cool atmosphere, keeping still, peace and quiet cold drinks	Warm stuffy rooms, movement stooping, coughing, eating, exertion and touch	Bryonia
	Headache brought on by bright lights or severe coughing fits	Resting with head elevated, cool rooms, skipping a meal, being left alone	Mental efforts, talking, noise, sunlight, touch, sympathy	Natrum mur
	'Morning after' headache with nausea and irritability	Gets better as day goes on, peace and quiet, warmth, sleep	First thing in the morning cold draughts, stress, being disturbed smoking	Nux vomica
	Head pain brought on by atmospheric changes, thunderstorms, hunger, fright or shock	Massage, eating, after a sound sleep, bathing face in cold water, cold drinks	Lying on painful side, shock, cold air, thunder and lightning, morning and evening, mental	Phosphorus

Which Homeopathic Remedy?

FOR PREGNANCY continued

Condition	Symptoms	What makes it better?	What makes it worse?	Suggested remedy
Heartburn	With flatulence and distension	Belching, cool air, fanning yourself coffee, milk, warm, damp weather	Evenings, after eating, fatty foods	Carbo veg
	Indigestion feels like a stone in your stomach, bitter regurgitation	Sleep, nap, heat, warmth, evening, wet applications, firm pressure	Morning on waking, after meals, coffee, alcohol, cold dry weather/winds, spices, overwork, anger, sedentary lifestyle, noise, 3am–4am, loss of sleep	Nux vomica
	Dyspepsia, no thirst	Open air, cold dry air, cold food, cool applications, pressure, gentle movement, sympathy, consolation	Heat and stuffy rooms, humidity too many clothes or bedclothes lying on the left side, eating rich or fatty foods emotional upset	Pulsatilla
Insomnia	Over-stimulated, thoughts crowd your mind	Warmth, lying down	Extreme emotions, noise, open air, cold	Coffea
	Difficulty falling asleep, restless, wakeful, too tired to sleep	Cool air, peace and quiet	Stress, heat	Passiflora
	Recurrent nightmares, disrupted sleep, muscle twitches, yawning	Being alone, deep, regular breathing, warmth, changing position	Emotional strain, shock, anxiety, coffee, chill, smoking	Ignatia

Condition	Symptoms	Worse for	Better for	Remedy
Miscarriage	Sudden red blood with fear of losing the baby	Cold dry wind, getting chilled, night, fright, shock, noise, light	Open air, rest, warm sweat	Aconite
	Blood loss with great exhaustion	Slight touch, draughts, cold fresh air, movement, night, esp. midnight, autumn, eating fruit or acid things	Firm pressure, warmth, sleep	China
	Profuse bleeding with nausea and vomiting bright red blood	Cold weather, excessive heat, damp weather	Firm pressure, open air rest	Ipecacuanha
	Blood loss from injury and accident	Gets worse as day goes on, heat, exposure to hot sun, rest, slightest touch, cold, damp, movement, exertion injuries, falls	On first getting out of bed, rest, lying down with head lower than feet	Arnica
Nausea	Nausea with hot or cold clammy perspiration, retching	Excessive heat, damp weather, after vomiting, movement, strong smells	Open air, cool conditions, rest, keeping still	Ipecacuanha
	Craves food but feel nauseous	Evenings, the smell of food, mental exertion, loss of sleep	Bending forward	Colchicum
	Vomiting frothy mucus, craving salt, thirsty	Late morning, hot atmospheres, dampness, mental exertion, emotions, sympathy, fatty or starchy food, noise, music, touch, pressure, full moon	Open air, cool bathing, sweating, rest, going without regular meals, peace and quiet, seashore	Natrum mur
	Vomiting, irritable, exhausted, indifferent, hot flushes	The smell of food, afternoon, cold, fasting, getting wet, storm brewing, touch, emotional demands of others	Exercise, keeping busy, elevating the legs, eating small amounts, fresh air	Sepia

Which Homeopathic Remedy?

IN LABOUR

Condition	Symptoms	What makes it better?	What makes it worse?	Suggested remedy
Overdue	Changeable moods, needs lots of sympathy, mild Braxton Hicks contractions but no progress, ambivalence about the birth	A good cry, attention, cool fresh air, gentle exercise	Stuffy rooms, warmth, rest, evening and night, lack of fresh air	Pulsatilla
	Restless and complaining; feels like the baby will never come	Eating	Noise, pain, anger	Cimicifuga
	False labour pains, exhaustion	Activity, gentle movement, perspiring, lying with head elevated	Brooding over events, being overheated, mid-morning	Gelsemium
	Pains come and go, feeling trapped, wants to escape	Left alone, head propped up, wrapped up snugly	Touch, noise, bright lights, movement	Belladonna
	Irritable, false pains, fretful and weak	Cool, fresh air	Cold, exhaustion	Caulophyllum
Painful	Labour progresses but is very painful, nervous and restless between contractions, back pain makes you cry out	Warmth, holding ice in the mouth lying down	Extremes of emotion, strong odours, night	Coffea
	Pain with distress, weakness, spasmodic, comes and goes	Being left in peace and quiet, warmth, being upright	Touching, too much light, moving around	Belladonna
	Tired and fretful near the end of labour, distressing back pains	A warm bed	Moving around	Causticum

	Symptoms	Better for	Worse for	Remedy
Painful continued	Can't bear the pain, cross, unreasonable, wants to get away from herself, thirsty	Cool fresh air	Noise, anger	Chammomilla
	Pain with a frequent urge to urinate or pass a stool	Sleep, nap, heat, warmth, evening, wet applications firm pressure	Getting chilled, eating, drugs, anger, 3am–4am, loss of sleep	Nux vomica
Slow progress	Irregular ineffective contractions, exhaustion, nausea	Cool fresh air	Cold	Caulophyllum
	Afraid of bieng alone, pains suddenly cease, irregular weak contractions	Company, fresh air, open air, cold dry air, cold food, cool applications, pressure, lying on the painful side, gentle movement, sympathy, consolation	Heat and stuffy rooms, emotional upset, humidity, too many clothes, lying on the left side, eating rich or fatty foods	Pulsatilla
	Bears down but has difficulty pushing the baby out, mother is very distressed	Being uncovered, rubbing, stretching out limbs	Heat, covers	Secale
	Contractions cease entirely, anticipates them with fear	Urinating, bending forward, movement, perspiring, lying with head elevated	Emotions, ordeals, stress, movement, heat, sunlight, smoking, hot, damp weather	Gelsemium
	Lots of rapid contractions but no progress, back pain, mother fears she or the baby will die	Rest, open air, warm sweat	Fright, night, cold dry wind, getting chilled, shock, noise, light	Aconite
	Emotions or external events disrupt labour, spasmodic pains	Resting with head elevated cool rooms, skipping a meal, being left alone	Mental efforts, talking, noise, sunlight, touch, sympathy	Natrum mur
	Contractions 15–30 minutes apart, ineffective, weak	Food, warmth and rest	Excitement, worry, mental and physical exertion, cold	Kali phos

CHAPTER 14

HYPNOTHERAPY

DEPRESSION
ANXIETY
FEAR
QUITTING SMOKING
REDUCING LABOUR PAINS
RESOLVING CHILDHOOD TRAUMAS
RELAXATION
HEADACHES
DIGESTIVE DIFFICULTIES
LOWERS BLOOD PRESSURE
REGULATES BREATHING
RELATIONSHIP DIFFICULTIES

☑ **Requires a professional therapist**
☑ **Suitable for self-treatment after instruction**

The power of suggestion can be strong medicine ...

It is also one of the oldest forms of therapy. Ancient writings confirm that the Sumerian priest-doctors used hypnotic suggestion as a therapeutic tool, as did the later Hindu fakirs, the Persian magi and the Indian yogi.

The Ebers papyrus tells us that ancient Egyptian priest-doctors would often ask those who consulted them to fix their gaze upon a glossy piece of metal to help induce a trance-like state in which healing could occur – a technique which is commonly used by modern practitioners. Today, hypnotherapy is considered so powerful that it has been used by dentists and doctors in lieu of an anaesthetic. There is even a case of a 15-year-old girl undergoing a heart operation while under hypnosis.

The mind is divided into two parts, the conscious and unconscious. Some practitioners liken it to an iceberg, with the conscious mind being the tip and the unconscious being the large mass which lies beneath the surface. We cannot live in the unconscious; it is too vast and complex. To function on a day-to-day basis we need to remain in the realm of consciousness. But this does not mean that we should ignore what is going on below the surface, since the conscious and unconscious mind are constantly interacting in subtle ways of which we are largely unaware. What lurks in the unconscious can often be at the root of our health problems and anxieties.

Hypnotherapy uses the power of suggestion to induce a trance-like state that enables individuals to explore the hidden levels of their minds and emotions. Positive suggestion can then be made and heard by the patient at a very deep level to help bring about change.

While some view hypnotherapy as an opportunity to shine a light on the dark corners of the mind, others find it a scary prospect, almost like having to walk down a dark, unfamiliar street in the dead of night. But the unconscious does not only hold our scariest, darkest secrets and memories. It also holds all of our potential for good, such as our underused creative talents and unexpressed emotions. Hypnotherapy, then, is a way to tap into the good as well as the unfamiliar and uncomfortable, in a safe, supportive space.

Among those who use hypnotherapy, more than 90 per cent will derive some benefit. Relief from stress is the most commonly reported effect, but it has been used to treat a wide range of conditions, including headache, respiratory problems, sleep disorders and chronic pain.

Under hypnosis, you enter a state of consciousness somewhere between sleeping and waking. Many of us have experienced this powerful state, for instance, at night when we are drifting off but have not yet fallen asleep. Some people experience this as a time when insight seems to come out of nowhere or when they suddenly recognize a solution to a problem which has been plaguing them for some time.

Hypnosis is not the same as sleep. When the brainwaves of hypnotized subjects have been monitored, an increase in alpha wave activity – the electrical impulses which are produced when humans are in a relaxed but mentally alert state – has been revealed. When a subject is asleep, slower delta waves are the predominant type of brainwave activity.

Hypnotherapy is also not the same as the stage hypnotism you see on TV. The common confusion between the two means that many people feel unable to take hypnotherapy seriously. Yet research continues to show that, under the right circumstances, hypnotherapy is a very powerful catalyst for change.

Unlike stage hypnotism, your therapist is not controlling your thoughts or making you act in a certain way. On the contrary, in hypnotherapy, you direct the course of the therapy. Your therapist is there to help you gain insight into your everyday actions, to achieve your goals and feel confident about the decisions you make. When an individual feels comfortable with their therapist, the benefits of increased relaxation and the control and management of pain can be very significant.

MESMERIZED

Modern hypnosis began in the eighteenth century with an Austrian doctor called Franz Anton Mesmer, who used a technique he called 'animal magnetism' to treat a variety of psychological and psychophysiological disorders such as hysterical blindness, paralysis, headaches and joint pains.

Mesmer was something of a showman and his experiments contributed to a widespread scepticism about the uses of hypnosis. He was, however, the source of a new word in the English language; the trance-like state of his patients came to be known as being 'mesmerized'.

In addition, for hypnosis to work you must have the desire to be hypnotized. Your willingness is what opens the door to a dialogue with your own subconscious. People who have lived with physical or emotional pain for years often forget what it is like to live without that pain. The pain becomes deeply ingrained as part of their personality. They may even believe, on some level, that they need their pain to make them feel alive. Hypnosis can take you back to a time when you were generally pain-free and help you to re-experience what that was like. It can provide positive, supportive suggestions which can help you create new patterns in your life. It can also help to free you from uncomfortable physical symptoms. For instance, if you are experiencing headaches as a response to stress, you can begin to build new, pain-free responses to help you deal with stress. Given this, it's perhaps not surprising that the overwhelming experience of hypnotherapy patients is one of relaxation and relief.

CAN ANYONE BE HYPNOTIZED?

Practitioners believe that 90 per cent of people can be helped into a hypnotic state. But research shows that around 4 per cent of the population is especially susceptible to entering a trance-like state, often without any outside help or suggestion. A person's susceptibility to a hypnotic suggestion may also be related to heightened states of confusion or emotion.

Under the right conditions, crowds of people can be hypnotized and, for instance, mass hypnosis of people by the Indian fakirs has been well-documented. During one such occurrence, a crowd believed they were watching the Indian rope trick. Later, photographs revealed that the rope had fallen and the fakir was just standing there doing nothing.

HYPNOTHERAPY IN PREGNANCY

Hypnotherapy has increasingly been the focus of several research trials and there is now a good deal of evidence to suggest that hypnosis, though it works primarily on the mind, induces a number of profound physical effects, namely a slower heart beat and breathing rate, dilation of the bronchi in the lungs, lowered blood pressure and more efficient production of stomach acid.

It is also thought that hypnotherapy can produce a positive change in immune system function, making it an appropriate tool for treating a range of health disorders. Because of this, hypnotherapy may be particularly suitable for those suffering from hypertension, asthma, recurrent headaches and nausea.

Hypnotherapy can either be performed with a practitioner or the method can be taught to individuals who can then practise self-hypnosis as either a preventative or cure. It can induce a profound sense of relaxation and some pregnant women find it a useful adjunct to other antenatal preparations. If you are feeling tense about the pregnancy or forthcoming birth, hypnotherapy can provide a safe structure in which to explore the root of your anxiety.

Hypnosis can also be used to address practical matters. Studies have shown it to be very useful in helping pregnant smokers to quit – indeed this is one of the most common reasons why pregnant women consult a hypnotherapist.

Insomnia, whether caused by stress or by physical discomfort, can also benefit from this form of therapy. Techniques learned in the consulting room can be used at bedtime, for example, to calm an over-active mind. To further encourage sleep, some therapists may also 'prescribe' the use of a relaxing spoken word or music tape to use before falling asleep.

Occasionally, nausea will respond well to hypnotherapy. This may be because stress can exacerbate symptoms of nausea or perhaps, in some cases, nausea may be a physical expression of some aspect of the pregnancy which the mother literally 'can't stomach'. Either way, hypnosis, especially if combined with changes in diet and lifestyle, may be beneficial.

Hypnotherapy in Labour

Studies have shown that women who use hypnotherapy antenatally and during labour feel a greater satisfaction with the process of labour and report other benefits such as reduction in anxiety and less fatigue. In addition, women who use hypnosis may have somewhat shorter labours than those who use conventional relaxation techniques, and may also use less medication and experience less depression after birth.

Hypnosis is also sometimes used to aid relaxation in labour. In one study published in the *Journal of the Royal College of General Practitioners*, hypnosis showed greater benefits during labour over the traditional relaxation technique, psychoprophylaxis (a form of progressive muscle relaxation). Compared to those women who did not have hypnosis, first-time mothers given hypnotherapy had labours which were more than 90 minutes shorter. For women having second and subsequent babies, labour time was reduced by around 40 minutes. The hypnosis group also reported greater satisfaction with the birth.

While we tend to think of it only as helping to reduce pain, hypnosis can be particularly useful in reducing labour complications. For instance, it may be helpful in turning babies into more favourable positions. When two groups of American women who were nearing the end of their pregnancies and whose babies were in the breech position were compared, twice as many babies in the hypnotherapy group turned spontaneously into the more favourable head-down position.

In this study, women were encouraged, during the hypnosis session, to relax but were also asked to tell the therapist why they thought their babies were in the breech position. Women with breech babies often report feeling as if their lives are upside down, and this study suggests that there is an emotional as well as physiological component to the position of a baby. Once the question of why the baby is upside down is answered to the mother's satisfaction, the baby often turns. Even if it doesn't turn, the mother may feel better able to accept that this is the way her baby has 'chosen' to be born.

All the available evidence suggests that women who use hypnotherapeutic techniques in labour tend to have fewer unnecessary interventions. For instance, in a study published in the *Journal of Women's Health* in 1993, self-hypnosis was taught to a group of 87 women, but not to 56 comparable women (called 'controls'), all of whom were under the care of the same doctor. After the outcomes of these two groups were compared, the hypnosis group was further compared with a second group of 352 low-risk women who gave birth at the same hospital but under the care of a different physician. Results showed that the women in the hypnosis group used significantly fewer epidurals – 11 per cent less than the controls and 18 per cent less than the second group of women. They also had 19 per cent fewer drips than both other groups and 12 per cent and 16 per cent fewer episiotomies than the control and second group, respectively. Also, 21 per cent more births took place in the labour room when compared with the control groups.

Hypnotherapy certainly seems to fulfil the criteria of a 'good' therapy – since it helps to equip the woman with the confidence and skills to help her cope with the enormous transition of pregnancy and birth.

WHAT TO EXPECT

Hypnotherapy usually takes place in a quiet room. Some therapists prefer to use dim lighting. At the first session, your therapist will ask you about your life, the reason why you have sought this particular therapy and what you hope to achieve through hypnotherapy. He or she will take a detailed case history. During this initial session, you will probably not have a therapeutic session but your therapist may try to induce a trance-like state to see how well you respond to hypnotic suggestion.

At the next session, you will be asked to sit or lie down – sometimes you are given a choice – and the therapist will help you into a hypnotic state. Sometimes he or she will do this by simply speaking quietly to you. At other times, you will be asked to fix your gaze on something in the room and focus on this until a change in your consciousness becomes evident.

You will probably have discussed beforehand what issues you would like to explore. While in this trance-like state, your therapist will ask you questions specific to these areas. For instance, if you wish to quit smoking, your therapist may ask you to talk about smoking, asking why you smoke and when you smoke. If smoking is a coping strategy, your therapist may begin exploring with you more positive ways to cope with stress and reinforce the positive message that your will-power is strong enough to make such a change.

If you are seeking to use hypnotherapy for pain relief, your therapy may consist of an exploration of what 'pain' means to you and may include positive reinforcing statements, such as 'my body will never give me more pain than I can cope with'. Your therapist will also spend some time teaching you simple self-hypnosis techniques which you can use during labour. Your therapist should, however, be honest with you about what can and cannot be achieved in this area. The success of such therapy depends, to some extent, on your own personality type. Some people are more susceptible to suggestion than others. In any case, hypnotherapy will not take the pain away, but can make you more confident of its effective management and its place in labour.

The British Hypnotherapy Association (*see* page 303) can help you find a qualified therapist in your area.

TAKE CARE

As with all forms of therapy, both conventional and alternative, the skill of the practitioner is everything. Although hypnotherapy employs several mechanical methods to help the client reach a state of altered consciousness, your therapist should not approach the business of hypnotherapy like a mechanic. Preferably, your therapist should have some training and skill in counselling or psychotherapy. You should be given an opportunity at the end of each session to talk about what you have experienced and integrate it into your everyday consciousness. You should feel fully supported emotionally and safe in the process of entering and emerging from this other consciousness, this 'other' side of yourself. Leaving the session with unresolved issues can make you feel worse, not better.

SELF-HYPNOSIS

If you are seeing a hypnotherapist, the chances are that he or she will give you some self-hypnosis suggestions which you can practise at home. These usually involve taking a few moments each day to relax and reinforce the positive suggestions which you will have received during your formal session.

Anyone can practise simple self-hypnosis at any time. You will need to be somewhere quiet where you can be assured of few distractions. You should be sitting comfortably in a chair. You should also be clear about what you would like to achieve, for instance, whether it is complete relaxation of your tense muscles, letting go of obsessive thoughts or steadying your nerves.

Begin by focusing on a point in front of you. It can be anything – a picture, a pattern on the wallpaper, a place where the light is reflected on the wall. Let everything except that object drop away from your mind. Stare at the object until you begin to see it change. That's the signal to close your eyes. Now let your attention come to your body. Identify some part of your body that you are particularly aware of at that moment. It could be your eyelids or the way your lungs are taking in air, it could even be your aching head. Let everything else drop away and focus on this place until you feel a change – your breathing may slow down, or a tense muscle may begin to relax.

Once you reach this stage, you can help yourself go into a deeper trance by counting slowly backwards from ten to zero. Some people like to imagine that they are descending a staircase and that with each step they are becoming more relaxed and receptive. Using the opposite method, counting up and ascending the staircase is a good, gentle way of coming out of hypnosis.

When you are in this trance-like state, find as many different ways of saying the same constructive things to yourself as you can. It may help to write out a few statements you can use during self-hypnosis beforehand. Try to keep these positive: instead of saying, 'I will not be tense,' say 'I am relaxed and calm.' Or instead of saying, 'I won't let the pressure get on top of me,' say 'I am coping well with all the things I have to do.'

Try also to make good use of your imagination. For instance, if you are tense about something you have to do at work, imagine yourself coping well and with confidence at each stage of the day; getting up, travelling to work, arriving at work, seeing your colleagues, taking meetings and so on. Let yourself explore all the possibilities of the day and your reactions to them, reminding yourself at each stage that you are coping in a relaxed and positive way.

Remember that negative patterns take a long time to build up and they can take an equally long time to knock down. Doing this type of exercise just once or twice is unlikely to produce great results. You will need to practise each day for a month or more to even begin to feel a change occurring in yourself and the way you respond to outside forces. Like many alternative therapies, hypnotherapy requires a commitment to yourself and your own well-being. It also requires a commitment of time in order to restructure the less constructive aspects of your personality and to bring out your best qualities.

CHAPTER 15

MASSAGE

WHAT IT'S BEST FOR

STRENGTHENS IMMUNE SYSTEM
IMPROVES CIRCULATION
LOWERS STRESS
LOWERS BLOOD PRESSURE
DEPRESSION
HEADACHES
CONSTIPATION
PREVENTS PERINEAL TRAUMA
STIMULATES LABOUR
ESTABLISHING INTIMATE CONTACT
REDUCES FEAR AND ANXIETY
SKIN CONDITION
REMOVE TOXINS FROM THE BODY
PROVIDES SENSORY STIMULATION FOR THE BABY

☑ **Requires a professional therapist**
☑ **Suitable for self-treatment after instruction**

Touch is a universal language – it comes from the heart but is spoken by the hands...

In days gone by, massage was an integral part of maternity care. Midwives were often local village healers and weekly, even daily, massage was common during pregnancy. It was also one of the main therapeutic tools and means of support in the immediate postnatal period. As technology began to command a central role in antenatal care, massage came to be seen as a 'luxury' by mothers and the people who cared for them. Until a few years ago it was almost unheard of as a legitimate therapy for pregnant women. The tide is turning, however, and the popularity of massage as a supportive therapy throughout pregnancy is once again increasing. A good massage can be good medicine, providing comfort, reducing pain and physical discomfort and enhancing feelings of well-being. Touch can also play a fundamental role during labour and massage therapists are in a unique position to offer skilled, tactile support at this time.

Although it has been practised for thousands of years and is an ancient relative of many modern types of body therapies, such as shiatsu, aromatherapy massage and reflexology, massage is a therapy almost by default. Quite apart from any therapeutic effect of the laying on of hands, comforting and sensitive touch, stroking and soothing, provide a profound form of spiritual nourishment for the body.

Holistic massage can create a sense of optimism, nurture self-acceptance and body awareness, lighten up the spirit and help the 'receiver' to let go, strip off the mask worn to face the world and get a better perspective on his or her true self.

Massage can be performed at home or by a professional therapist; each has its own unique advantages. Going to a professional therapist can become a part of your life, helping you to establish a regular nurturing routine for yourself. Receiving a massage from, or giving a massage to, your partner can be a way of establishing and maintaining deeper intimacy during pregnancy and beyond.

The same techniques which are used in general massage, Swedish massage, deep pressure-point massage, and reflexology can be incorporated into pregnancy massage. While loving intention is probably more important than expert technique, some approaches, particularly in labour when a

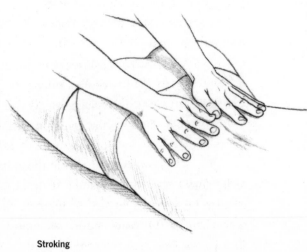

Stroking

mother's skin is highly sensitive, can produce better results than others. These are:

Stroking

Using the flat of the hand, fingertips or thumbs to create flowing, relaxing movements. Stroking is sometimes likened to performing a ballet on the skin, so let yourself be creative. Using a variety of different strokes in combination is usually most effective, thus strokes can be light or firm, straight or circular, brisk or slow. Stroking is usually done in the direction of the heart, except on the legs, where stroking down from the thigh to the feet will provide the sensation of removing tension. When working on the head and face, stroke upwards, taking tension out of the top of the head. Stroking aids circulation, calms the emotions and tones the muscles.

Kneading

This involves, grasping the flesh between the thumbs and fingers in a flowing motion from one hand to another. It is particularly effective on the shoulders, hips and thighs but can also be used on other fleshy parts of the body to relax muscles, aid circulation and to encourage excretion of toxic build-up. If the muscles are very tense, knead briefly and move on to another area. Keep returning briefly to the tense area until it begins to loosen up.

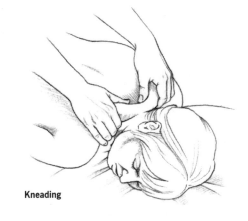

Kneading

Pressure

Use fingers and thumbs to work directly on specific muscles. Using small, circular movements may be beneficial and very pleasurable,

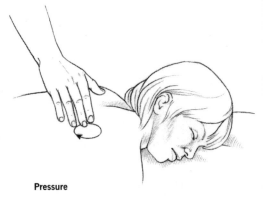

Pressure

especially on either side of the spine during a back massage. The knuckles can also be used effectively to apply a wider area of firm pressure.

Percussion

This is the name used for a variety of techniques such as cupping, hacking and pummelling (as in Swedish massage). These techniques are appropriate on the fleshy,

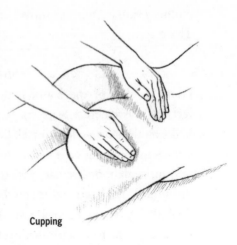

Cupping

muscular areas of the body in order to stimulate and improve circulation. They are stimulating and should be avoided if the mother is stressed out and requires a relaxing massage.

The environment of the massage is also important. Those elements which make a massage a more relaxing experience include:

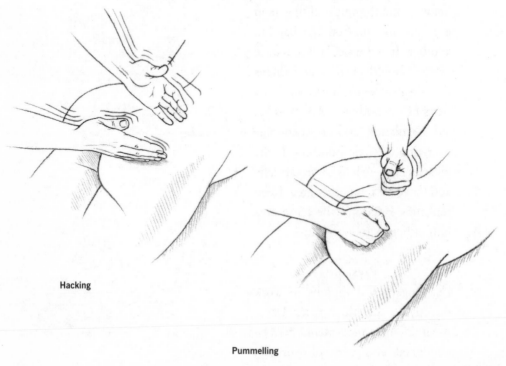

Hacking

Pummelling

• a room that is warm, peaceful and, if you prefer, softly lit

• a firm, but padded surface. A futon is ideal but a floor padded with towels and blankets and covered with a sheet is also suitable.

• towels to cover the receiver and pillows to support her body (especially important for pregnant women). In late pregnancy you should avoid lying flat on your back when receiving a massage. Instead, lie supported by pillows or on your side.

• massage oils are pleasant, but not always necessary.

• the giver should have short fingernails, clean hands and no watch, bracelets or rings.

GUIDELINES FOR 'GIVERS'

If you are new to massage, here are a few guidelines to help turn simple massage into an effective way of easing some of the common complaints your partner may experience during pregnancy:

Headaches Keep your touch firm, but caring. Gently circle the temples and jaw muscles and massage the whole of the scalp with your fingertips, working upwards, to disperse pain and constriction. Stroke across the forehead, gently pressing on the inner and outer corners of the eyes and lightly pinching along the ridge of the eyebrows. As tension in the neck and shoulders is often a contributory factor, working these areas may also be helpful. Don't forget to massage the ears – there are many acupressure points on the ears which benefit all parts of the body.

Aching neck and shoulders Your partner should be sitting up and well-supported. Work the shoulders first. Moving outwards from the neck, use your whole hand to knead the muscles on the top of the shoulders. Make small circles on either side of the spine between the shoulder blades with your thumbs. After loosening up the shoulders, move on to kneading, stroking and circling the back of the neck and pressing along the base of the skull.

Backache The woman should be on her side or leaning forward over a bean bag or birth ball. Using long, gliding strokes, work upwards along the long muscles on each side of the spine. Follow this by circling outward with the palms of the hands. Small, spiralling circles with the thumbs will help loosen tight spots. With one hand on top of the other make slow, deep circles over the base of the spine and the sacrum. Squeezing and kneading the buttocks and hips will also help to relieve tension.

Aching legs The woman can be on her side or propped up with her back well-supported. Long, gliding strokes from ankle to the top of the thigh, and back again, will help to release the lactic acid which can build up in muscles after long hours of standing or vigorous exercise. Use firmer pressure on the up-stroke, lighter on the way down. Follow this with gentle, draining strokes pushing upwards with alternate hands. Long, gentle strokes beginning at the ankle and moving up the inner thigh and back down the outer thigh can also be very relaxing.

Insomnia Try a gentle massage last thing at night when the woman is already in bed. Using gentle, soothing strokes on the back, feet or face for as little as 15 minutes can create a state of deep relaxation.

Cramp Start by stretching the limb (perhaps by walking around if it's a leg cramp). A firm massage of the muscle groups involved will encourage them to loosen and release. Friction (rubbing the skin in quick, light motions) will help bring circulation back to the area.

MASSAGE IN PREGNANCY

The biggest benefit of massage is the way in which it stimulates the immune system and helps to combat anxiety and depression. Massage during pregnancy can also create a sense of body awareness and even be used to increase your tolerance to pain. Some practitioners use deep-tissue massage to mimic the common patterns of uterine contractions. To do this they apply moderate pressure to certain areas of the body, gradually increasing the pressure, then peaking and gradually diminishing the intensity of the massage.

While this is happening, the woman can focus on her breathing and become skilled at releasing herself into sensations which originate and change outside of her conscious control. Doulas in America are increasingly offering women in their care the option of this type of massage as a form of prenatal preparation. Some women report that it is more effective than the exercises they are given in antenatal classes.

Self-massage can also have benefits. Numerous studies report that massaging the perineum, inside and out, every day from about 32 weeks reduces the risk of tearing and the rate of episiotomy. This form of intimate massage can be performed by the woman on her own, or by her partner.

MASSAGE IN LABOUR

Simple self-massage can also be used to stimulate labour. Several studies show that breast and nipple massage can reduce the number of pregnancies managed as 'post-dates' by as much as two-thirds.

The level of pain a woman feels in labour may also be reduced through massage therapy. Massaged mothers generally report a decrease in depressed mood, anxiety and pain, and show less agitation and anxiety during labour. In addition, there is evidence to suggest that massaged mothers experience significantly shorter labours, shorter hospital stays and less depression postnatally.

The best person to massage a woman in labour is the person who is most in tune with her individual experience and needs. This may be her partner, but equally it may be a close friend or even her mother. A woman in labour may want a lot of touching or none at all and her needs may change from moment to moment during the course of labour. Every woman's needs are different, but as a general rule rubbing, stroking and kneading are more effective during the first stage of labour, and during the lull between contractions.

Massage during labour is most effective when it follows the rhythm of the woman's breathing. As the contraction builds, the giver should use upward strokes on the in-breath, and downward strokes on the out-breath. Only when the contraction has begun to abate can the giver begin to direct the rhythm of the massage using gentle, calming strokes to help the woman regain her equilibrium.

Massaging a woman during labour is an expression of love and responsibility. Many women report feeling totally lost and abandoned when their partners, for whatever reason, abandon the task of massage as labour progresses. When a giver brings the same level focus and commitment to his (or her) role that the woman brings to the job of birthing her baby, birth can become a genuinely shared and fulfilling experience.

During the second stage, many women prefer the feel of a firm, warm palm, fist or forearm. Compression and counter-pressure are effective in alleviating a backache labour once the mother finds a comfortable position to labour in. The person who is giving the massage may wish to employ techniques from shiatsu, reflexology or acupressure to help combat nausea, anxiety and pain during labour. Most massage techniques can be applied in or out of water, and many women find the combination of hydrotherapy – using a water pool, shower spray or bath – and massage therapy very effective during labour.

What to Expect

A good holistic massage therapist will want to establish some understanding of who you are, what is important to you and what your immediate and long-term needs are. Your initial consultation may involve a process of answering questions about all these things. In addition, your therapist will want to know how far along your pregnancy is, whether you have suffered any physical complaints so far, what your previous experience of pregnancy was, if any. You will have a full body massage in the first session.

Follow-up treatments, which usually last 45 minutes to an hour, will build on what comes out of this first session. Your therapist will 'listen' to your body and sense how it reacts, for instance, whether you tense up when touched in certain places, the noises you make as the massage progresses and any feedback you have after the session and at the beginning of the next.

An effective body massage is difficult to give even through light clothing, so you will generally be asked to strip off your clothes and lie down, either on the floor or a special mattress or a massage table. Your therapist will cover with a towel those parts of your body which are not being worked on. The towel will be repositioned as he or she works along your body. Some therapists use massage oil and some do not, often according to their client's wishes.

TAKE CARE

'Beauty' massage is not the same as therapeutic, holistic massage. Do check that your therapist is a qualified masseuse with a full knowledge of the physiology of the pregnant woman and what is appropriate in labour and birth. During the first trimester only the lightest of touches is appropriate and, as with all forms of massage, there are certain manoeuvres which should not be performed and areas which should not be massaged during pregnancy. During the first trimester, abdominal and sacral massage are probably best avoided, particularly in women who are prone to miscarriage.

There are times when it is inadvisable to apply a home treatment. Use your common sense and don't work over broken skin, or sites of infection, inflammation or swelling, since you run the risk of spreading infection to other areas of the body. Massaging varicose veins can release clots into the circulation and should be avoided. You should also seek advice if you feel you may have torn a ligament or tendon, or if you feel that you have pulled a muscle or put your back out. In such cases, lay massage, however loving its intent, may only make the condition worse. Always seek professional advice if you are in acute pain.

Also be aware that massage can evoke powerful feelings in the receiver. Our bodies often 'hold', or store, emotional pain within the muscle tissues. Before beginning treatment with a professional therapist, you may want to discuss their views on this 'holding' and whether they are sufficiently trained in basic counselling skills to help you talk about any feelings which come up during treatment. You should never have to leave a massage session feeling strung out, upset and unsupported.

FETAL MASSAGE

When you are pregnant intimacy takes on a new definition. While we often view massage as something which one person gives to another, there is another form of massage which helps to expand the concept of intimacy into the realm of a family affair.

Fetal massage is a relatively new technique in which both parents make time each day (usually upon waking or before going to sleep) to be with the baby. During this time you should not talk; instead spend time silently caressing each other and the woman's belly.

Babies know when they are consciously included in their parents' lives. So, when you have finished stroking, spend some time talking about the baby, about the things which you are doing to prepare for his or her arrival and your dreams and hopes for the future. Or you can talk about your relationship, what you are feeling and your concerns for the future.

Intimacy requires practice, so even if you feel awkward at first about including the baby in such intimate moments, try to stay with it. The way that a child is nurtured in the womb and the way it experiences life during this influential period will influence its future physical and psychological health and the way the child goes on to lead its life. Expressing and experiencing feelings of love and sexuality, not just through sexual intercourse, but through caressing, fondling and massaging, release beneficial hormones into the mother's blood system. These chemical messengers send out clear and life-enhancing signals to the baby: *you are loved.*

CHAPTER 16

NUTRITIONAL THERAPY

WHAT IT'S BEST FOR

IDENTIFYING NUTRITIONAL DEFICIENCIES
DIAGNOSING ALLERGIES
PRE-ECLAMPSIA
GESTATIONAL DIABETES
ANAEMIA
PROMOTING FETAL GROWTH
NAUSEA
FATIGUE
PREVENTING BIRTH DEFECTS
CONSTIPATION
REDUCING THE RISK OF MISCARRIAGE
SUPPORTS THE IMMUNE SYSTEM
PROMOTES HEALTHY SKIN, HAIR AND BONES

☑ **Some conditions require a professional therapist**
☑ **Some conditions are suitable for simple self-treatment**

Let food be your medicine and medicine your food ...

This is one of the earliest dicta of medical care. Today we know that many of the diseases which plague our modern society have their roots in what we eat, and what we don't eat. For instance, a 1997 report by the American Institute of Cancer Research confirmed that between 30 and 40 per cent of all cancers in the West are directly related to our modern diets, which are generally low in complex carbohydrates, fresh fruits and vegetables, and high in fat, salt and additives.

In recent years, the field of nutritional medicine, with its emphasis on correcting nutritional imbalance and detecting food sensitivity, has grown in stature. This is in part because of our increasing awareness that many chronic health conditions can be self-inflicted, sometimes resulting from a combination of unhealthy lifestyles and unfriendly environments. It is also a response to the growing list of unacceptable side-effects which accompany the drugs (both prescription and over-the-counter) which we use to suppress the symptoms of chronic illness. During pregnancy you may find that you are more acutely aware of the potential risks to your baby of taking even so much as a decongestant or an indigestion tablet. Given this, many women who feel the need for a safe alternative which can produce long-term results turn to nutritional medicine.

Nutritional medicine is not the same as healthy eating, however. Healthy eating guidelines are general recommendations for the general population. They do not take into account the fact that each of us has different constitutional strengths and weaknesses. What might be an adequate intake of iron, zinc or calcium in one person, for instance, may not be adequate in another. The main aim of nutritional medicine is to identify individual weaknesses and deficiencies and their causes and correct these through the use of supplements and the appropriate selection of foods.

In addition to identifying nutritional needs, a nutritional therapist will also pay close attention to other aspects of a person's life, such as the impact of potential allergens.

ALLERGY OR INTOLERANCE?

Food sensitivity can take many forms, the most usual being an allergy or an intolerance. The two terms are often used interchangeably but the distinction is important. An allergy is a reaction to a food or other substance which causes an immune system response. Often (though not always) this response can be measured with immunological blood testing. To confuse matters, some experts believe that a person can be allergic to a substance without producing measurable antibodies. An intolerance is a reaction to a food which does not cause an immune system reaction (or at least a measurable reaction) but which still causes adverse physical symptoms.

Surprisingly there is often little difference in the external physical symptoms, such as skin rashes or respiratory problems, which you may experience, though an allergic response can be much more intense than one caused by intolerance.

THE IMPACT OF ALLERGIES

When the poet Lucretius said 'one man's meat is another man's poison' he could have been talking about allergies. We still do not know why, for instance, one food or substance should cause an allergic reaction in one individual but not in another. What we do know is that food sensitivities, including allergies, are a major cause of chronic disease. Over the last few decades the number of allergic reactions that have been identified has grown enormously. There is scientific literature identifying more than 1,700 separate studies which link food sensitivity alone to certain mental symptoms such as depression and schizophrenia. Clinical papers have also linked food intolerance with Crohn's disease, irritable bowel syndrome, asthma, arthritis, eczema, migraines, hyperactivity and even epilepsy. Many nutritional therapists know this, and the diagnosis of potential allergies is an important part of their treatment.

When you eat something to which you are allergic, your body reacts as if it has been invaded by an alien organism and employs all its defences. Your immune system goes on full alert and a series of complex chemical chain reactions take place. Antibodies which fight off the offending substance are produced and histamine, one of the chemicals which produces symptoms such as breathing difficulties, loose bowels and inflammation, is released. Eventually, the toxic by-products of this biochemical war must be excreted from your system, putting your liver and kidneys under increasing strain. Since the skin is one of the major excretory organs of the body, skin rashes can also be the result of the body's attempts to get rid of these toxic by-products.

Some women find that during pregnancy new symptoms such as skin reactions, sinusitis or an increase in asthmatic symptoms occur. Given the increased load which your vital organs must carry, this is not surprising. However, if your body is carrying an additional toxic load, because of an allergic reaction to food or in reaction to allergens in your environment, your health may deteriorate.

Despite the accumulating evidence, many conventional doctors are sceptical about the link between allergies and illness. Some are also quick to dispute, often without justification, the curative potential of nutritional supplements. So if you suspect that a particular food or something in your environment may be your 'poison', you may have to seek the assistance of a qualified nutritional therapist to help you confirm your hunch.

THE QUESTION OF SUPPLEMENTS

Nutritional supplements are a mainstay of nutritional medicine. In a perfect world all our essential nutrients would come from food. But we all know that this is not a perfect world and that the idea of a perfect diet is a myth. Also, as individuals, we are more than the sum total of what we eat. Outside factors such as the amount of stress we are under, whether we live in heavily polluted areas and what medications we are taking or have taken, will all affect how well we absorb and use the nutrients gained from our diets.

A nutritional therapist will always try to use supplements in appropriate ways and in appropriate amounts. This is in complete contrast to the practice of most antenatal clinics, where the tendency is to dole out single nutritional supplements in isolation and irrespective of the individual woman's needs. For instance, just giving a woman an iron tablet may not help boost her blood iron levels. Her problem may not be iron intake but iron absorption. What the woman may really need is a boost in her vitamin C intake, either through supplements or by simply having a glass of citrus juice with her meals. In addition, excessive iron supplementation can deplete the body of another essential nutrient, zinc. Another example is calcium. Calcium absorption is aided by the presence of other minerals, especially zinc and magnesium. During pregnancy, it may be wise to confront the magic bullet mentality which plagues our society and remember that taking any kind of pills, even vitamins, can turn you into a patient.

Very little research exists on the nutritional requirements of healthy pregnant women. But what little there is suggests that there is folly in mega-dosing or taking supplements just in case.

Studies have shown that mega-doses of vitamin A (retinol) may cause birth defects (ironically, deficiency in this vitamin can cause the same thing). The levels which are implicated, however, more than 20,000 to 30,000iu daily, are beyond what most women will ever take. Also, not all forms of vitamin A are implicated. Beta carotene, a naturally occurring substance which converts into vitamin A in the body, appears to be safe. Nevertheless, it is probably wise not to exceed recommended doses for this nutrient during pregnancy (*see* table, page 237).

Perhaps the biggest example of nutritional magic bullets, however, is the advice that all pregnant women should take folic acid. There is good evidence that in high-risk women, taking 400ug/mcg of folic acid preconceptually and during the first two months of pregnancy may lower the risk of the baby developing spina bifida. The problem is that there is no way of accurately addressing the question of who is at risk and who is not. In Britain, for example, rates of spina bifida are unusually high, suggesting an as yet unidentified environmental link rather than something inherently wrong with the baby-making equipment of British women. Nevertheless, folic acid has been seized upon as a kind of cure-all, with some women taking it for insurance purposes long after they are supposed to and long after it has been shown to be effective. With whole ranges of food being fortified with extra folic acid, a new question arises: can we get too much of a good thing?

Nobody knows, but continuing research from Hungary suggests that there may be problems with folic acid overdosing. The Hungarian researchers believe that the 'protective' effect of folic acid may be indirect. Instead of preventing neural tube defects from occurring, they suggest it works by increasing the rate of spontaneous miscarriage. If this is true then it has important implications for women who are prone to miscarriage. Such women may be told that they are miscarrying because the baby was in some way abnormal (though there is seldom evidence to support this view). They may even be taking higher doses of folic acid in order to prevent the alleged abnormality from occurring again, unaware that supplementation may represent a case of swings and roundabouts.

On the plus side, there appears to be some truth in the idea that many women are deficient in certain nutrients which are relevant to their reproductive health. One of these is zinc. Low levels of zinc have been found in women who have recurrent stillbirths and miscarriages, though it is not clear why this should be so. One theory is that women who have recurrent stillbirths may have extremely high levels of the toxic metals cadmium and lead. Zinc is known to protect against both these elements and aid their excretion from the body. Moderate supplementation may be a reasonable course of action.

Given the deficiencies in many of our diets, it is not unreasonable, and unlikely to be dangerous, for a woman to consider taking a good-quality multi-vitamin and multi-mineral supplement during pregnancy (remembering that this is there to supplement, not replace, a good-quality diet). In this context, 'good quality' means a supplement which is free from unnecessary additives and which contains natural complexes such as rice bran, sprouted barley juice, alfalfa – all of which aid the absorption of vitamins into your system. Taking your vitamins with nutritious food, the original 'natural complex', can often aid their absorption and utilization.

Multi-vitamins rarely contain enough of vitamins C and B-complex and during pregnancy these are particularly important. If you are considering taking folic acid it is probably best to take it as part of a B-complex so that it may work more efficiently with other members of its 'family'.

If your multi doesn't supply around a gram of vitamin C, consider taking another supplement to make up the numbers. One gram a day of vitamin C is generally considered a nutritional minimum and there are many good-quality studies to show that this amount can prevent illness or (should you become ill) lessen its severity and duration. Vitamin C is also a 'complex' and is absorbed best when the supplement includes bioflavonoids and other synergistic compounds such as rosehips.

Women who are vegetarians will need to pay special attention to their diets and make sure that levels of zinc, B-complex, calcium and magnesium are all adequate. For vegetarian women, including dairy products in your diet will be helpful even if you don't normally do this, otherwise you may need to resort to supplements.

Also, do not make the mistake of thinking that what is right for one individual or culture is right for every individual and culture. What you need in terms of nutrition will vary according to where you live and what ethnic group you belong to. A good example of this is that women with dark skin, particularly if they are city dwellers, tend to be more prone to vitamin D deficiency during pregnancy. Supplementing with 400iu of D and 500 to 1,000mg of calcium daily may be appropriate in these circumstances.

If you have had unexplained previous problems in pregnancy, you may wish to consider having yourself tested either for vitamin and mineral deficiency or for high levels of toxic metals. The group Foresight can help with this (*see* page 303).

NUTRITIONAL THERAPY FOR PREGNANCY

Nutritional medicine has greatly improved our knowledge of the way in which nutritional deficiency contributes to ill health during pregnancy. Looked at from a nutritional point of view, many of the common symptoms of pregnancy are really a signal from your body to pay attention to how much, or how little, of the essential foods and nutrients it is receiving. There is a wealth of research on this subject, most of it linking unpleasant symptoms to a deficiency of some sort.

Reading through the list below, consider whether you are getting enough nutrients to sustain good health during pregnancy. You may wish to adjust your diet to include the foods suggested in the list on page 240, or to take the supplements to the recommended levels on page 237. These recommendations are, however, general. If you feel you need extra help, consult a qualified nutritionist who will be able to advise you and monitor your progress.

Anaemia

There's more to anaemia than simply low iron levels. A woman is said to be anaemic when her level of red blood cells falls below a certain point. Iron works with other nutrients in the body to increase red blood cell production and low levels of red blood cells can be the result of deficiency in B12, folic acid, manganese, copper and B6. Vitamin C helps aid the absorption of iron in the body, so consider supplements or take a glass of citrus juice with your meal. If you do resort to an iron tablet, make sure it is the more easily absorbed ferrous, not ferric, form. Look for preparations which include ferrous glucamate, ferrous flumerate and especially ferrous bisglycinate. You are unlikely to need more than 40 to 60mg of elemental iron daily.

Candida

This condition, which causes thrush, is strongly linked to diet. Apart from the suggestions in chapter 2 you should make sure you are getting enough vitamins A, B-complex and C as well as the minerals zinc, iron and magnesium, since a deficiency of these may predispose you to attacks from fungi. If you must take antibiotics, make sure you also take pro-biotics in the form of acidophilous and bifidobacteria to help counter their harmful effect on the body's 'friendly' bacteria and minimize the chances of opportunistic fungi taking hold again.

Many conditions in pregnancy benefit from extra B6. However it may be wise to observe a small caution during the last trimester of pregnancy. B6 at levels above 100mg may (in some women) interfere with the production of prolactin, the hormone necessary to produce breastmilk. For those intending to breastfeed, it is a good idea to keep supplemental B6 between 25 and 50mg during this time to ensure adequate production of milk for your child.

Carpal Tunnel Syndrome

This uncomfortable condition, the result of extra accumulated water putting pressure on the nerves in the wrist (known as the Carpal Tunnel), responds well to 100mg daily supplements of B6.

Constipation

A change of diet and plenty of water and exercise are still the best way to deal with constipation. However, increasing your intake of vitamin C may also help to alleviate the condition. Aim to include at least one gram (1,000mg) daily.

Gestational Diabetes

This is not the same as pre-existing diabetes and is likely to be caused by a temporary change in your metabolism during pregnancy. In particular, vitamins of the B-complex family may be needed to help bring your body back into balance. Studies show that 100mg of B6 daily can bring about a great improvement in this condition.

Haemorrhoids and Varicose Veins

Extra supplements of vitamin C, 1–2 grams per day, and vitamin E up to 800iu daily can be effective. Taking essential fatty acids such as those found in fish oils or evening primrose oil will also maintain a healthy circulation. Follow the general advice in chapter 2 for avoiding constipation.

Insomnia

Inability to fall asleep or remain asleep is often related to stress. Because stress takes its toll on the body's nutritional supplies try taking calcium, 100mg daily, together with magnesium, 200–500mg daily – the combination may produce a tranquillizing effect. Stress can deplete levels of B-vitamins, so supplement with a B-complex which includes 50–100mg of the entire family. If you have trouble maintaining sleep it may be because of night-time hypoglycaemia (a sudden drop in blood sugar in the night). Make sure your supplement has adequate levels of nicotinamide (also known as niacinamide or B3) and take it before bedtime. Don't megadose, as nicotinamide can place a strain on your liver in high doses. Unless otherwise directed, and under the consultation of a qualified nutritionist, use it only as part of a B-complex.

Nausea

During pregnancy your needs for B6, B12, folic acid, zinc and iron will all increase. Adequate amounts of these nutrients are probably enough to ward off the nausea associated with pregnancy. Therefore, if you are feeling very ill early in pregnancy, in addition to your minimum of 400mcg daily of folic acid, extra supplements of B6 in the region of 100mg daily may be needed. You may also require B12 in 50ug/mcg daily doses. Symptoms should usually disappear within a week or two, in which case you should consider halving your dose. Zinc deficiency is also implicated in pregnancy nausea – aim for 20mg daily.

Pre-Eclampsia

Apart from careful attention to diet, and investigating the contribution of food allergies to her condition, a woman who has pre-eclampsia should consider increasing her intake of certain important nutrients. Chief among these are B6, calcium and magnesium. On their own, none of these nutrients has been consistently shown to help pre-eclampsia. However, supplementing with all three, especially if combined with an improved diet, may help prevent the condition from appearing, and may prevent a worsening of your condition (or even improve it) if it has already appeared. Vitamin B6 should be taken in doses of 10 to 50mg daily; calcium 1,000mg daily and magnesium 400–600mg daily. There is also research to suggest that supplemental vitamin E may improve pre-eclampsia. It is especially important to take pre-eclampsia seriously and take action at the first signs of its appearance.

Premature Labour

If you have had a previous premature labour or are experiencing early contractions, it may be a sign that you are deficient in certain essentials such as magnesium and calcium. Taking 1–2g of calcium in the form of calcium gluconate or amino acid chelate per day combined with magnesium, 500–800mg daily, may help. Also consider taking 2–3g of evening primrose oil daily. Always consult your doctor if you experience signs of premature labour.

Restless Legs

This uncomfortable sensation in the legs, rather like an electric shock which makes you jittery and unable to sit or lie still, may be due to folate deficiency. In addition to any B-complex you may be taking, try increasing your intake of vitamin E. There is evidence to show that doses of around 300iu daily taken for around three months can be effective. Iron and magnesium deficiency may also come into play, so make sure you are getting optimum levels of both.

Stretch Marks

If your skin is giving way under the strain it may be a sign of zinc deficiency. Vitamins C and E are also necessary components of healthy skin. Applying vitamin E cream to the abdomen during the last few weeks of pregnancy may also help maintain your skin's elasticity.

HOW MUCH IS ENOUGH?

At the risk of giving yourself a pregnancy-related headache, it is worth taking a closer look at any multi-vitamin supplement you are taking to check if you are getting optimum levels of all the essential nutrients.

If yours is lacking, first consider altering your diet to include more foods rich in the missing nutrients. Only if this is impossible, or if there are pressing reasons why you might consider a supplement such as unrelenting nausea, should you include more supplemental nutrients in your regime. The optimum levels for the essential nutrients during pregnancy are as follows:

Vitamins	Optimum levels	Minerals	Optimum levels
A	5000–7500iu	Calcium	1000–1500mg
D	400–500iu	Phosphorus	1200mg
E	100–300iu	Magnesium	400–700mg
C	500–2000mg	Iron	30–60mg
B1	25mg	Zinc	10–30mg
B2	25mg	Sodium	3000mg
B5	50mg	Potassium	5000mg
B6	50100mg	Manganese	5mg
B12	50–100ug/mcg	Selenium	25mg
Folic acid	400–800ug/mcg	Iodine	175mg
Niacin (B3)	50mg		
Biotin	200mg		

WHAT TO EXPECT

When you first visit a nutritional therapist you will be expected to answer some very detailed questions about your diet. Many find this a little daunting. Eating has become so automatic to so many of us that we can barely remember what we ate for breakfast, let alone what we have eaten over the last week or month. To help get a good picture of what you eat, your therapist may ask you to keep a food diary, noting down what you eat and any physical symptoms you experience.

Uncomfortable symptoms which you experience fairly soon after eating one type of food are not always a reliable indicator of allergy or intolerance. Sometimes they are coincidental – an allergic response may take many hours to surface after eating the offending food. Some therapists may refer you for blood tests, others prefer the elimination diet as a means of identifying foods which may or may not cause an adverse reaction. Pregnancy is not a time to go on a strict elimination diet, so your therapist should work with you to identify as closely as possible the main potential allergens and remove a select few of these from your diet.

Although the process of eliminating foods temporarily and then reintroducing them may sound a bit haphazard, it is probably just as accurate as going for extensive, and expensive, blood tests. First of all the accuracy of such tests is hotly disputed. The ones which are within the reach of most pocketbooks tend to look for only one or two 'markers' (chemicals present in the blood which indicate an allergic response) in the blood. The most accurate ones use several different markers, but can also be prohibitively expensive.

Such tests are further confounded by the fact that a food to which you are intolerant may produce a symptom but may not necessarily produce an antibody response which can be measured in your blood.

If your therapist favours the elimination diet, he or she will probably recommend that you take some of the most common food allergens out of your diet. These include wheat, citrus, dairy, egg, corn and soya. Your therapist may also suggest you investigate environmental allergens such as dust mites, the gases given off by plastics, cookers and heating appliances, perfumes and cleaning chemicals, since these can also cause adverse reactions.

Some nutritional therapists have an interest in Oriental medicine. This means that in making a diagnosis and recommendations they will try to balance your food intake in terms of yin and yang. This means striving for a harmony between sweet and sour, cold and hot and expansive and contractive foods. The choice of foods may seem eccentric at first and may even be at odds with what you have been taught about 'good' food. Nevertheless, outstanding results can be produced by following such regimes.

Several groups provide nutritional advice and put people in touch with competent therapists. These include the British Association of Nutritional Therapists, the Register of Nutritional Therapists, the Society for Promotion of Nutritional Therapy and the Institute for Optimum Nutrition as well as the British Society of Allergy, Environmental and Nutritional Medicine (*see* pages 302–3).

GOT TO HAVE IT?

Food cravings and aversions are a normal part of life, but seem to become intensified during pregnancy. While aversions can be difficult to explain, cravings have come under much scrutiny over the years. Often the craving is not for the food itself, but for what it contains and the effect it has on your body. Equally, a craving can be the result of a dietary imbalance; diets which are high in grains often produce wild cravings in some individuals. A craving is not a bad thing, it's a message from your body. If you are sufficiently in tune, you will be able to respond to it appropriately. If a craving is allowed to turn into a binge, however, it can exacerbate existing imbalances. Most of us find it easy to give in to cravings for chocolate and other sweet treats, but too much sugar is certainly not good for you and can drastically lower your immunity. This is just one reason why it may be helpful to try to understand where cravings come from and the best ways to deal with them.

Annemarie Colbin, American nutritionist and founder of the Institute for Food and Health, combines Western and Eastern perspectives in her work. Over the years she has identified three main reasons for cravings: addiction/allergy, discharge and imbalance.

Addiction and allergy are two sides of the same coin. They both produce psychological or physiological symptoms which can be temporarily suppressed by eating the longed-for food. Eating the food makes the person feel better, though it does not cure the underlying problem.

Discharge is the term for a person who has changed their diet and is experiencing a longing for a food which is no longer part of their regime. When you alter your diet, for instance changing from a diet high in processed foods to a raw food diet, the body begins to release, or discharge, toxins as well as the chemical 'memory' of these foods. The body may interpret this chemical memory as need, even though it is not a genuine craving. That is why, when you do eat the longed-for food, it isn't as satisfying as it might be.

Imbalance is another very common problem created by modern diets. In a fast-moving world we tend to grab quick foods and often our diets are very high in one particular sort of food, usually carbohydrates, at the expense of others. Since the primary aim of the body is equilibrium, a craving for a particular food or foods can be seen as the body's attempt to restore balance. In particular, a craving for fats and sweets together, such as those contained in baked goods and ice-creams, may be a signal of protein deficiency. Pregnant women take note, since adequate protein intake is very important during this time.

To diminish or eliminate a craving, use the information on the following list adapted from Ms Colbin's excellent book, *Food and Healing* (*see* Bibliography).

In addition, American nutritionist Earl Mindell believes that these common cravings may signal the need for an increase in specific nutrients:

Cravings

Peanut butter/nuts B-vitamins, protein and fat. You need more of each when you are pregnant. A good quality supplement will help diminish the craving and will be lower in calories!

Olives, pickles Sodium – your pregnant body needs more of it.

Bananas Potassium which helps to maintain the body's water balance and normalize the heart beat.

Cheese Calcium, phosphorus and aluminium. Eat more broccoli as a lower-fat alternative.

Apples Calcium, magnesium, phosphorus, potassium. In addition, if you have a high-fat diet, your body may be craving the pectin for its ability to lower cholesterol.

Cantaloupe Potassium and vitamin A are its main nutrients. But it also contains vitamin C, calcium, magnesium, phosphorous, biotin, and inositol – so it's not a bad craving to give in to.

Milk Calcium is the obvious choice. But milk also contains useful amino acids such as tryptophan, leucine and lysine. As long as you're not allergic, let yourself have the odd extra glass.

Eggs Full of protein but also sulphur, amino acids, selenium and, in the yoke, fat. The white, by the way contains useful fat, dissolving choline which is why the humble egg is considered a first-class protein meal.

Finally, some women experience uncontrollable cravings for chocolate while they are pregnant. Chocolate is a complex food, the consumption of which begins a complex series of biochemical reactions in the body. Cravings for chocolate need to be addressed on both the physical and emotional levels. Eating chocolate may stimulate the release of 'feel-good' brain chemicals (called neurotransmitters) in the body; this combined with the immediate sugar boost may help a woman who is tired or depressed to feel better, albeit for a short time. Most commercially produced chocolate, however, is laced with pesticides, additives and other undesirable synthetic chemicals (many of which are not listed on the label). A more positive approach to feeling good would be to pursue a regular course of exercise and relaxation and, if necessary, consulting a therapist to deal with feelings of depression and lack of self-worth. Chocolate also contains magnesium and iron, so another tactic is to make sure you are getting enough of these through your daily diet.

At the other end of the scale, as long as your diet contains a wide variety of foods, the odd aversion is unlikely to cause nutritional deficiencies. However, if you suddenly develop an aversion to what for you is a major source of nutrients, make sure you substitute other foods which will make up the deficit. For instance, it is not uncommon for women to develop an aversion to red meat during pregnancy. As long as you are eating plenty of other protein foods (fish, cheese, nuts, tofu) and leafy green vegetables you will still be getting the iron and protein you require.

Eliminate a Craving

Craving	Consider	Eat more	Eat less	Try instead
Sugar (for example cakes, pastries, biscuits, sweets and ice-cream)	Restrict your intake or eliminate it completely	Whole grains, baked yams, squash, apples, dates, cooked fruit	Meat, salt, dairy	Frozen bananas instead of ice-cream, desserts sweetened with barley malt, rice syrup, maple syrup
Salt	Limiting your intake	Seaweed, black beans, vegetables	Sweets, fats, alcohol, meat, grains	Natural soy sauce, miso (in small amounts), herbs and spices
Milk products	Cutting down or eliminating it completely	Leafy greens, whole grains, beans, fish	Sugar, baked goods, fruit, meat	Tofu (in small amounts), nut milk
Fats and sweets (including baked goods made with natural sweeteners, whole wheat flour and oils)	Limiting your intake	Proteins such as beans, fish, chicken, eggs	Grains, fruit, salad	None
Coffee	Cutting it out of your diet	Vegetables, salad	Salt, acid forming foods such as meat, sugar, flour, grain	Grain coffee, herbal teas
Alcohol	Cut down or eliminate it completely	Complex carbohydrates, vegetables, corn, leafy bitter greens	Fats, salt, miso, soy sauce, animal protein	Non-alcoholic beer, fruit juices, herbal teas

CHAPTER 17

OSTEOPATHY AND CHIROPRACTIC

WHAT IT'S BEST FOR

BACK PAIN

IMPROVING POSTURE

LOW ENERGY

JOINT PAIN

MUSCLE RELAXATION

REALIGNING/SUPPORTING THE SPINE

NECK AND SHOULDER PAIN

OEDEMA

HEADACHES

BLADDER FREQUENCY

MORNING SICKNESS

IMPROVING CIRCULATION

INDIGESTION AND HEARTBURN

☑ **Requires a professional therapist**

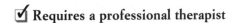

Not every alternative therapy has its roots in the mysterious East …

Both osteopathy and chiropractic emerged in the West, a little over 100 years ago. Both evolved from the 'bone setters' of developing America and began life with a rather more mechanistic view of the body, although many practitioners in both disciplines now take a much more holistic approach than their rustic predecessors.

Osteopathic and chiropractic therapists would probably agree that the spine is the bearer of the mother and her child. During pregnancy, some of the most profound physical changes you experience will take place along your spine. For instance, as pregnancy progresses, the combined weight of your growing baby and uterus can significantly alter the curvature of your spine. You may begin to feel pain, particularly in the lower back but also in the buttocks and down the legs.

Later in pregnancy, hormonal changes soften the bones and ligaments in the pelvis and elsewhere, increasing their flexibility during labour. This flexibility, however, makes the pelvis more unstable and less able to bear your weight. Being upright becomes increasingly difficult and you may feel a more insistent pain in the lower back and legs as time goes by.

Back pain is a common complaint of pregnancy but not one for which you must simply suffer in silence. The subtle alignments which an osteopath or chiropractor will be able to make in your back can help your body cope better with the increasing pressure on the whole spinal structure. Also, there is some evidence that, because the spine is connected via multiple pathways to all the organs of the body, dealing with back pain during pregnancy may cure some other common symptoms in pregnancy as well as helping to avert potential problems in labour, such as painful backache and poor positioning of the baby.

Cervical curve

Thoracic curve

Intervertebral discs

Lumbar curve

Sacral curve

The Spinal Curves

OSTEOPATHY

Osteopathy is a system of diagnosis and therapy which was devised by an American doctor, Andrew Still, in the late 1800s. Still was an engineer, so not surprisingly he developed an early interest in the body as a machine. He was also an army surgeon whose experience taught him just how brutal the conventional medicine of the day could be. Spurred on by the fact that three of his children died from spinal meningitis, he began to explore more compassionate ways of approaching the prevention of disease and the maintenance of health.

Dr Still quickly became convinced that the body was a self-regulating, self-healing organism. He was among the first to stress the importance of the structure of the body in relation to its function. Good health, in his view, was the result of the joints being properly aligned and, he believed, the spine played a vital role in supporting the whole structure of the body, linking not only joints but muscles as well. When any of these systems was out of alignment, he reasoned, illness was the likely result. Although radical for its time, Still's theory was not entirely new. The ancient Greeks and Romans also appreciated the role of the spine in our overall health and well-being.

Other practitioners, such as William Garner Sutherland, took Still's ideas and refined them. Sutherland, in particular, is credited with proving – in spite of medical scepticism – that the body, even the bony skull, is in a constant, dynamic state of motion and our tissues, organs and bones have a unique pulse and expand and contract in a harmonious rhythmic impulse.

Osteopathy spread from America to Britain in the early 1900s. Today it is a flourishing and well-respected system of physical therapy. In the UK osteopathy is the only alternative therapy to be accorded the status of a statutorily self-regulated profession.

The musculo-skeletal system influences the body mainly through the nervous system, which permeates the entire body and whose function depends partly on the unhindered flow of nerve impulses and blood. We now know that nerves don't just transport electrical impulses; they also transport fats, proteins and other essential cell substances. This goes some way towards explaining why it is so important to our continued good health that the musculo-skeletal system is functioning properly.

During pregnancy, the spine and joints come under pressure. There will be extra strain on the back, knees and hips due to the extra weight you are carrying. Because of the softening of the ligaments, certain parts of the body become more vulnerable than others. Strain and compression can lead to aches and pains commonly felt in the lower back, hips and pelvis. An osteopath can maintain the alignment of your body and keep joints mobile through gentle manipulation, reducing pain and helping to readjust your centre of gravity so that the body remains a relatively stable, self-supporting structure.

Although primarily viewed as a therapy for back and neck problems, osteopathy has a good track record in treating a wide range of other common problems. Today, a great many osteopaths see their role as encompassing somewhat more than just a mechanistic view of the body. Many are also trained in naturopathy and approach the body as a holistic system. Apart from joint manipulation, osteopaths believe that soft-tissue manipulation can help improve the flow of vital energy in the body, in much the same way as acupuncture. Thus, osteopathy takes on a much wider role during pregnancy and may be used to resolve digestive disturbances, low-energy, asthma, circulatory problems, headache and many other uncomfortable complaints.

In addition to soft-tissue manipulation, rhythmic mobilization of the joints and sometimes more forceful movement of the joints, osteopathy can also work through the head to treat a number of disorders. This is called cranial osteopathy. Comparing the skills of a cranial osteopath to osteopathy in the rest of the body is rather like comparing the skills of a watchmaker to those of a car manufacturer. Cranial work is precise and gentle, providing maximum benefit with minimum input. This is what makes it particularly suitable, for instance, for babies. By gently manipulating specific areas of the skull and upper neck, your practitioner will be able to feel the pulse, or energy, of the membranes, cerebrospinal fluid and brain (which are different from the pulse of the blood) and use these to make a 'diagnosis' and as a guide to appropriate treatment.

THE PROBLEM WITH BIPEDS

It has been argued that the human animal is poorly adapted to its upright posture. In bipeds – that is, two-footed animals – the discs and joints of the spine have become weight-bearing, but they were originally intended to be slung underneath a horizontal back. The stomach and the pelvic contents, including the diaphragm, sag easily, which can contribute to health problems such as constipation, hernia and hypertension. In our upright position, the heart and much of the circulatory system must work against gravity and the air passage of the lungs must drain upwards by coughing and sneezing.

Adding insult to injury, we don't use our bodies in a healthy way. We sit at desks all day, performing small, repetitive movements over long periods of time. Women, in particular, wear restrictive clothing and high heels which prevent free movement. Certain body states such as obesity, pregnancy and emotional stress, which make the muscles tense up, only add further strain, affecting almost every area of the body.

For these reasons, when an osteopath treats your aching back, he or she is not simply treating your back.

CHIROPRACTIC

Chiropractic places even more emphasis on the spine than osteopathy. Chiropractors will often use X-rays and other conventional diagnostic tools to help them reach a diagnosis and will generally treat all perceived disorders through spinal manipulation. The treatment is more robust than in osteopathy and can involve sharp, thrusting movements. Chiropractic aims to put things back in place: to adjust bad posture, restore function of the spinal and pelvic joints and correct any interference with the nervous system caused by deviation in the spinal and pelvic alignment.

Most people go to a chiropractor because of back and neck pain. As a therapy it also has a good track record for easing headaches. Individuals who have sustained an injury from a fall or car accident, even if it occurred long ago, also report a reduction in pain with chiropractic therapy. At the time of writing, chiropractic was on the verge of joining osteopathy in becoming a statutorily self-regulating profession in the UK.

Like osteopathy, there can be a wide range of practice among chiropractors. Some prefer to work just on the spine whereas others take a more holistic view of the body, believing that simply focusing on the mechanics of the spine means losing the original aim of the therapy. These latter therapists will treat the spine and extremities and give counsel on diet and lifestyle in order to treat the whole person. Some liken their practice to that of the homeopath, using significant information on the mental, emotional and spiritual symptoms to make a more comprehensive diagnosis of the individual's needs. Not all chiropractors take this view, however, so it might be wise to spend some time talking to individual therapists to find out what their philosophy of health is.

HEARING IS BELIEVING

The first documented chiropractic adjustment was performed in 1895. A janitor in the building where Daniel David Palmer, the 'founder' of chiropractic, worked had been deaf for 17 years. He lost his hearing when, while stooping to pick something up, he felt something give way in his back and immediately became deaf. Palmer reasoned that the deafness was due to this back injury and could be restored by reversing the process. A relatively simple adjustment to a misaligned vertebra in the janitor's neck restored his hearing completely.

SPINAL MANIPULATION IN PREGNANCY AND LABOUR

Both osteopathy and chiropractic can, in theory, be used to treat the same range of symptoms. In practice, however, around 90 per cent of those individuals consulting a chiropractor tend to be suffering mainly from back, shoulder and neck complaints. Osteopaths tend to see those with a wider range of physical and emotional complaints. Whom you consult may also be related to where you live. In the UK, osteopathy is the more common practice, while in the US chiropractic is surpassed only by general practice in the number of available practitioners.

When your spine is in proper alignment you may find that many other niggling complaints begin to disappear. Both osteopathy and chiropractic have been shown to be effective, for instance, in the treatment of chronic headaches. Chiropractic, in particular, has proved as effective as pain-relieving drugs and produces better long-term relief without the side-effects. Chiropractic has also been shown to help eliminate pain and the need for bed rest in women suffering from back pain during the later stages of pregnancy.

Both therapies are safe for the unborn child and many women find them a useful and relaxing adjunct to normal care during pregnancy.

There is research to suggest that women who receive spinal manipulation during pregnancy have a much lower reported incidence of back pain during labour. Osteopathy has been reported to significantly reduce both fetal and maternal fatalities as well as difficult labours. One reason for this may be that when the spine and pelvis are in alignment, the baby has more room to settle into a favourable position in preparation for birth. Thus both therapies may be useful for the mother whose baby is in a breech or posterior position.

WHAT TO EXPECT

During your initial appointment, your practitioner will take a detailed case history, including information about your lifestyle, work, diet and any medical conditions you have suffered from. Information about your pregnancy, such as when the baby is due, what kind of birth you intend to have, any previous pregnancies or miscarriages or any problems in previous pregnancies, will also be necessary.

You do not need to be in pain to consult an osteopath or chiropractor. It is reasonable to consult them for advice and reassurance or as part of a holistic 'well-woman' approach to pregnancy.

During your treatment, you may occasionally be asked to undress to your underwear. Your practitioner will want to see how you stand, checking spinal curves and posture and how your weight is distributed. You may be asked to move your arms, bend your legs or bend forward so that your practitioner can judge the range of movement in each of your joints. Your sitting posture will also be observed. Once all this is done, your practitioner will have a good picture of what parts of your body need treatment. Because your body will be changing throughout pregnancy, new changes should be taken into account before each session.

Subsequent sessions will involve different techniques. The osteopath may use soft-tissue manipulation, joint mobilization techniques or friction to improve local circulation and occasionally a high-velocity thrust to mobilize a very stubborn joint. The chiropractor will check the condition of your neck and spine and make adjustments and/or work to bring greater mobility to the joints according to his or her diagnosis.

Sessions usually last half an hour and treatment may be weekly, bi-monthly or monthly, depending on what is appropriate to your condition.

Early in pregnancy you may be given treatment while lying on your back or sitting up. As pregnancy progresses, treatment may take place with you lying on your side, sometimes with your abdomen supported by a pillow. Occasionally treatment may be given while the woman is sitting up. On request, your practitioner can also show your partner certain pain-relieving techniques. So from about 34 weeks on, ask your therapist if he or she can come along to learn how best to help you during labour.

Take Care

There are very few side-effects and contraindications for treatment with either chiropractic or osteopathy. However, you should probably not consider these forms of treatment if you:

• have a history of miscarriage or have had a threatened miscarriage
• have an inflammatory condition
• have an active pathology, such as a viral or bacterial infection
• have a history of joint hypermobility.

Chiropractic, more than osteopathy, has been the subject of several legal cases in which overly forceful movements were alleged to have caused damage to the spine. Because individual practitioners can vary in their approaches, be selective about who you choose as your therapist. Forceful manipulation is not really appropriate during pregnancy.

REFLEXOLOGY

☑ **Some conditions require a professional therapist**
☑ **Some conditions are suitable for simple self-treatment after instruction**

Being pregnant makes you more aware of your feet ...

Gradually, high-heeled shoes will feel less comfortable. Your increasing weight may be putting more pressure on your feet, making your arches feel sore. Standing for long periods of time can become increasingly difficult and at the end of a long day your legs, ankles and feet may feel swollen, hot and itchy. If the idea of a good foot massage sounds appealing, reflexology may be for you.

Reflexology, sometimes called reflex zone therapy, is a particularly sophisticated form of foot massage which has its roots in an Ancient

Chinese therapy and makes use of pressure points and energy pathways similar to those used in acupuncture and acupressure. Until fairly recently there was very little written about this type of therapy, but there is evidence that other ancient civilizations understood the interaction between the feet and the rest of the body. For instance, certain African tribes practised some form of foot therapy and Ancient Egyptian tomb paintings depict scenes of what appear to be foot massage.

The practice of reflexology re-emerged in Western culture in the early 1920s when an American ear, nose and throat doctor, William Fitzgerald, found that by applying pressure to a certain area of the foot he was able to anaesthetize the ear, enabling him to perform minor operations without an anaesthetic. After discovering that certain Native American tribes used a similar technique he refined his views further, using pressure on certain other foot points to alter his patients' perceptions of pain.

His research led him to divide the body into ten longitudinal zones running from the head to the toes and fingers (he called this zone therapy – a term still used by some practitioners today). At this time the feet had not yet been singled out as the optimum place for therapy, so the hands and the tongue were also used. Eventually word of this new technique spread throughout the US and the UK and practitioners were rediscovering and refining their own techniques.

Reflexologists believe that the soles of the feet, when viewed together, represent a map of the entire body. Reading the map of the body in reflexology is fairly simple. The right foot represents the right side of the body and the left foot the left side. The reflexes, or pressure points, which are stimulated are mostly on the soles of the feet, although there are a few on the top and sides of the feet as well. The reflexologist will draw an imaginary line across the middle of the feet representing the waistline. The big toes will represent the head, the little toes the sinuses and the heart point is found in the left foot, just above the waistline.

Through stimulating the feet the reflexologist aims to stimulate the body's own healing powers and its ability to rebalance itself. Although it is not a diagnostic tool, it is possible for the reflexologist to detect areas of disorder or disease which may be present in the body. Some may even

The Reflexes Chart

Right sole   **Left sole**

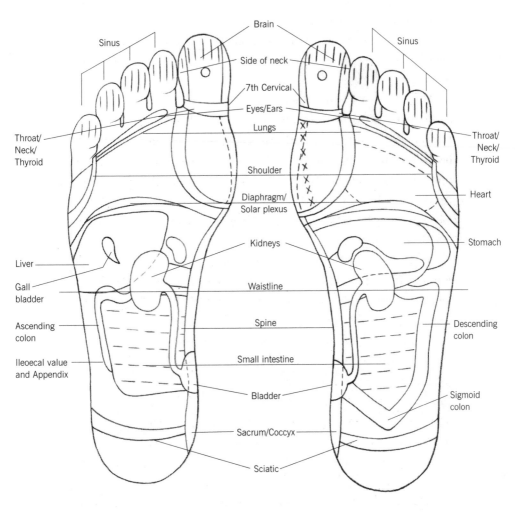

Sinus
Sinus

Brain
Side of neck
7th Cervical
Eyes/Ears
Lungs

Throat/
Neck/
Thyroid

Throat/
Neck/
Thyroid

Shoulder

Heart

Diaphragm/
Solar plexus

Liver

Stomach

Gall
bladder

Kidneys

Waistline

Ascending
colon

Spine

Descending
colon

Ileocecal value
and Appendix

Small intestine

Bladder

Sigmoid
colon

Sacrum/Coccyx

Sciatic

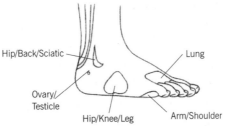

Hip/Back/Sciatic

Lung

Ovary/
Testicle

Hip/Knee/Leg

Arm/Shoulder

be able to detect areas of weakness in the body where future problems may arise. By massaging and applying pressure to these points, change can be brought about in the corresponding area of the body. This change could be to increase circulation to that part of the body or to a specific organ or to reduce nervous tension. It can also provide general stimulation to the healing energy of the body, helping to improve immune system function.

Similar reflex points to those found in the feet are also found in the hands. However, the feet are normally used because the reflex points are larger. Also, the fact that feet are protected day-to-day in socks and shoes means they are more receptive to massage. For self-treatment, however, hands can be very useful. Some reflexologists will also make use of cross-reflexes, that is, links between certain areas of the body. Thus, if you are experiencing pain in the hip, your reflexologist may choose to stimulate a point on your shoulder.

While some therapists still hold to Fitzgerald's zone theory, others see reflexology as a Western way of interpreting and understanding the Chinese meridians and their energetic connections to the rest of the body.

METAMORPHOSIS

A related therapy to reflexology is called metamorphic therapy, which makes use of the Oriental principle that certain parts of the feet correspond to life in the womb. Practitioners of metamorphic technique believe that massaging each foot with a vibratory motion along a line stretching from the big toe to the heel on the inner side of the foot can help heal any physical and emotional traumas which occurred in the womb. Although originally developed to help handi-capped children, this gentle technique can be used by anyone and might be supportive to those considering rebirthing (see page 167).

REFLEXOLOGY IN PREGNANCY

Research into reflexology is, at present, very thin on the ground. Much of what we know about its uses in pregnancy and labour come from therapists themselves, particularly midwife/practitioners who employ reflexology as part of their repertory of care.

In pregnancy, conditions such as nausea (particularly if it is associated with hormonal fluctuations), vomiting, oedema and heartburn respond well to reflexology. Practitioners also claim good results with constipation, both before and after birth. Although a qualified therapist may address constipation by stimulating the liver zone, you can produce good results at home by gently massaging your arches rather than attempting to duplicate a more complex technique. Varicosities, particularly haemorrhoids, before and after birth, can also be treated successfully.

Certain emotional states such as anxiety will also respond to stimulation of reflex points. During therapy, a mother may be encouraged to discuss her fears and worries and relax into the rhythm of the massage. With the aid of reflexology, the mother may find she begins to sleep better and that her body becomes gradually strengthened against the debilitating effects of stress and anxiety.

REFLEXOLOGY IN LABOUR

In theory, labour can be initiated by stimulating the reflex points relating to the pituitary gland and uterus. Labour can be accelerated in the same way. However, there is very little research to say how effective such stimulation can be.

Midwife/practitioners report being able to use reflexology to harmonize uterine action, either by strengthening and co-ordinating inefficient contractions or helping to reduce excessively strong ones. If the mother is hyperventilating, stimulating the solar plexus zone can help to regulate breathing, particularly in the second stage.

Pain in labour can be reduced by gentle work all over the feet, paying particular attention to the reflex zones for the uterus and other pelvic organs, the pituitary gland and lymphatic system. Even if your labour partner is not confident in his or her reflexology skills, a simple foot massage will serve to warm the feet, providing a beneficial boost to the spirits since many labouring women literally suffer from 'cold feet' as their energy and blood is directed elsewhere.

WHAT TO EXPECT

During treatment, which lasts about 45 minutes, both feet will be massaged in order to treat and support the whole body. Areas which appear to be tender are given the most attention and normally these areas will be less tender after treatment. It will probably not be possible to relieve all the tenderness in any one area with just one treatment. So, as a general rule, you should consider a course of six to eight treatments to begin to see real change. Long-standing health problems will, of course, take longer to treat.

Most people leave the reflexologist feeling re-energized and with a sense of well-being. Some, however, will feel more tired than before the treatment. It is also possible that reflexology will promote a healing reaction in some which may include skin rashes, the need to go to the toilet more frequently, or a cold. Some symptoms may temporarily worsen before they get better. This sort of reaction should not last for more than a week. Often it is a sign of the body trying to rid itself of toxins released during the massage.

The Institute of Complementary Medicine and the British Reflexology Association hold lists of qualified reflexologists.

TAKE CARE

It is important that you are seen by a practitioner who is experienced in working with pregnant women, since there are certain points which should not be stimulated during pregnancy or which should be approached with extra care.

Some conditions in pregnancy, such as placenta praevia (where the placenta covers the cervix) and placental abruption (where the placenta begins to peel prematurely away from the uterine wall) contraindicate the use of reflexology. Care should also be taken with those with a possible ectopic pregnancy, threatened abortion, fever and/or infection and any unstable pregnancy about which the therapist may be unsure. Although there is a good argument that miscarriage is a reaction of the body, not a reaction to reflexology, great care should be taken with those who are prone to miscarriage.

Reflexology is also usually contraindicated in cases of pre-eclampsia, although a regular massage incorporating gentle, harmonizing strokes may help to lower blood pressure enough to prevent mild pre-eclampsia from developing into a more severe form of the disease. If the woman has any form of bladder or kidney disease, caution should also be exercised. Only the most experienced of therapists should attempt to treat conditions such as cystitis, for instance, since there is a risk of spreading infection to other vulnerable areas of the urinary tract.

CHAPTER 19

SHIATSU AND ACUPRESSURE

WHAT IT'S BEST FOR

CARPAL TUNNEL SYNDROME
CONSTIPATION
HAEMORRHOIDS
CRAMPS
HEARTBURN
FATIGUE
BREATHLESSNESS
FREQUENT URINATION
INCREASED VAGINAL DISCHARGE
INSOMNIA
NAUSEA AND VOMITING
FLUID RETENTION
BACK PAIN
HEADACHE
INDUCTION/AUGMENTATION OF LABOUR
PAIN RELIEF

☑ Some conditions require a professional therapist
☑ Some conditions are suitable for simple self-treatment
after instruction

The ancient East and the modern West meet in today's practice of shiatsu ...

Perhaps this is why shiatsu is sometimes described as Japanese physiotherapy. Although this description is helpful to Westerners, it only partly illustrates the benefits of this wonderfully effective form of massage and manipulation. Shiatsu is a Japanese word made up of two written characters meaning finger (shi) and pressure (atsu). This ancient form of massage evolved from an even earlier form of massage called anma, which was brought into Japan from China (where it was known as amma) as early as the sixth century. The Japanese adapted the principles of amma while still adhering to the basic tenets of Oriental healing. Anma was used in conjunction with acupuncture and healing herbs, as well as lifestyle modifications, in order to encourage health.

It wasn't until the 1960s that shiatsu was recognized in Japan as an entity in itself, separate from anma. The shiatsu which we know today is still evolving, becoming a mixture of East and West as well as a kind of individual form of expression by its many practitioners. Typically, modern shiatsu involves many different kinds of pressure applied with the practitioner's fingers, palms, elbows and knees. Shiatsu has much in common with acupressure, since it also stimulates acupoints with pressure. But it is also different since pressure is sometimes applied to other areas as well.

In common with other Oriental therapies, shiatsu works on the flow of energy in the body, which in Japanese is called ki. In shiatsu, touch is used to assess the flow and distribution of ki in the body. Once assessed, your practitioner can then begin to aid the process of restoring balance. Some doctors may dismiss this as mumbo jumbo, but research in Japan has shown that the energy channels or meridians which are used in shiatsu (and which are similar to those used in acupuncture) lie in the connective tissues. The connective tissues form a continuum throughout the body; all the important body systems – circulatory, nervous, musculo-skeletal, digestive and other major organs – are sheathed in it. Every movement of the body, no matter how small, creates bioelectric signals (in other words, energy) which run through the connective tissue. Some points on the body generate more electricity than others. In Oriental medicine these are known as tsubos. Pressure on the tsubos generates small electric currents which are then conducted along specific pathways away from their point of origin.

But pressure is not the only technique used. Shiatsu also involves gentle stretching and manipulation techniques, perhaps the result of Western influence. A therapist may press, hook, roll, sweep, shake, rotate, pat, pluck, lift, pinch and brush. Even so, there are differences between shiatsu and, say, Swedish massage. For instance, while a Swedish massage therapist may use long, sweeping movements, shiatsu practitioners apply light, rhythmic movements and gentle but increasing pressure to meridians and sensitive pressure points. Sometimes the practitioner will 'hold' a hand over an area until he or she can feel a change. Often a hand may be passed over an area without touching it, either to heal or assess that area.

What they do all have in common is touch. All living things need to be touched and shiatsu helps to fulfil this need. It is the caring touch so characteristic of shiatsu which helps to trigger the self-healing process.

In addition, shiatsu is widely perceived to be a spiritual practice as well. Part of the training of a shiatsu practitioner is an ongoing commitment to self-awareness and development. After all, it can be very difficult to help balance someone else when you are burned out and unbalanced yourself. Shiatsu is also unique among massage therapies in that there is often a meaningful interaction between the therapist and the client (usually thought of as the giver and receiver). Benefits for the receiver include more body awareness, a greater feeling of integration between body and mind, and a deeper sense of connection with your baby and your own creative and reproductive powers, but also with the creative powers of the universe.

SHIATSU IN PREGNANCY

Because pregnancy can be a very emotional time, physical touch can be very reassuring and calming. So many women report feeling that touch is greatly missing elsewhere in their lives. Deep, sensitive massage is one way to help such women feel a sense of connection to another person. Also, while pregnancy is largely a state of health, we shouldn't take good health for granted at this time. Women's lives are busier than ever these days and unless the body's needs for rest, food and recuperation are met, a state of health can easily turn into a state of chronic disorder. For some, the demands of pregnancy combined with common hormonal changes mean that they often feel tired and vaguely ill long after the baby comes.

Shiatsu can help boost your vital energy and prevent such problems.

In Oriental medicine, kidney, spleen and stomach energy can become easily depleted. It is important to understand that in this system these organs are thought to have a much wider influence on the body than in Western medicine. For instance, the kidney is thought to be the primary source of energy for the fetus and will become affected almost from the moment of conception. When a woman works too hard and does not eat properly or rest well, a variety of symptoms connected to the kidney may appear. These include lower backache, oedema, fatigue, breathlessness, chronic coughs, anxiety, insomnia, vaginitis and cystitis.

The spleen, with help from the stomach, is responsible for producing blood, which nourishes your baby throughout pregnancy. After pregnancy, blood helps make breastmilk. Keeping the spleen toned therefore helps produce nourishing blood and healthy blood means a healthy baby. Imbalances of spleen and stomach can manifest as constipation, muscle spasms and cramps, haemorrhoids, heartburn, nausea, vomiting and oedema.

SHIATSU IN LABOUR

If you are experiencing a slow labour or you are overdue, or even if you are simply stressed about labour, shiatsu can help. You may wish to discuss labour with your practitioner, since he or she will be able to suggest ways in which you can work together to make it a better experience. Since your hospital may not encourage the presence of your alternative practitioner at the birth, you should consider having your practitioner teach your birth partner some simple techniques to help. If you are going to have more than one birth partner, choose the one whom you feel will be most in tune with your body and most able to deliver an effective massage.

WHAT TO EXPECT

There are many different styles of shiatsu, all of which are valid and effective. Many practitioners employ an eclectic mix of styles. A qualified practitioner will take a full case history and then make a diagnosis before treatment. There are as many different styles of diagnosis as there are styles of treatment. Some very experienced practitioners may palpate the abdomen or 'hara' in order to assess the relative energy in each of the internal organs. Other practitioners may take pulses. Whatever the styles of diagnosis, they are still based on traditional Oriental medicine and are all looking for energy

Your first session will last approximately 1 to 1½ hours and will include history-taking, some form of diagnosis and massage. Subsequent sessions will last approximately 40 to 50 minutes. Most treatments are given with the person lying down, fully clothed on a thin mattress or futon. Be sure to wear loose, comfortable clothing.

After each session you should be given a chance to talk about feelings which came up during the massage and discuss with your practitioner how to help maintain the sense of balance between sessions. The benefits of shiatsu are greatly enhanced when the receiver takes some responsibility for her body in this way.

After shiatsu treatment a sense of well-being is common. However, some people experience other effects. Because of the deep relaxation which shiatsu encourages and the stimulus to the major body systems, you may experience some 'healing reactions'. These are generally transient and can include coughing, mild headache, chilliness, aches and pains or tiredness and unexpected emotions. These symptoms are often a sign that the body is rebalancing itself and should disappear with each successive treatment, so any persistent symptoms such as headache and nausea should be investigated by your doctor or midwife.

Additionally, some people who are described as being 'out of touch' with their bodies do not benefit immediately from shiatsu. Such people may only be aware that something is wrong when there is a pain; more subtle body symptoms, which arose before the pain became chronic, tend to pass them by. For them, the sometimes subtle beneficial effects of shiatsu may also be missed. Sometimes, however, failure to feel any benefit from the therapy can be due to the practitioner's lack of skill as well as the fact that Shiatsu is not a therapy which suits everybody. When choosing a therapy, it is best to try to suit the therapy to the personality. When the match is good, health will improve.

Occasionally, very overweight people do not feel any immediate benefit. Deposits of fat around the internal organs occasionally form a barrier to ki. Shiatsu will be of some benefit but it can be hard for your practitioner to get the ki moving. Remember that pregnant is not the same as fat, but for women who are very overweight and pregnant, shiatsu is best combined with lifestyle modifications in order to maximize its benefit. The Shiatsu Society (*see* page 301) can help you find a practitioner in your area.

TAKE CARE

There are very few contraindications for shiatsu in pregnancy. Some practitioners believe that shiatsu is not appropriate during the first trimester. Certainly, your practitioner should avoid putting pressure on some points, and work on your lower back and sacrum should always be gentle. Certain areas on the lower leg should be avoided during the first trimester. If you have a history of miscarriage or there are signs of an imminent miscarriage you should avoid shiatsu.

In general, shiatsu should not be practised on those who have:

- a high fever
- just eaten – leave two hours after meals
- varicose veins – pressure should not be applied directly
- a history of high blood pressure
- a history of stroke or brain haemorrhage
- blood-borne cancer.

ACUPRESSURE

If you are drawn to the philosophy of acupuncture but dislike needles, you may find that acupressure suits your needs just as well. Acupressure is a non-invasive form of acupuncture which uses the same meridians and vital points. In order to help the body balance its energies, the acupressure therapist will use finger pressure, heat or cold to stimulate acupuncture points, or tsubos, on the body.

Tsubos are different from other areas on the body in that they have more neuroreceptors and conduct more electricity. Oriental practitioners would say that these are the points on the body where the Qi flows very near to the surface of the body. A sensitive practitioner will be able to feel this flow of energy at each tsubo. Firm pressure and non-damaging heat and cold applied to a tsubo can change the energy which flows from that point through the spinal cord and into the brain.

Acupressure can be done through most types of clothing, but for most acupressure techniques it is best to work directly on clean, dry skin. It can be a part of regular, formal therapy or you can apply it as a self-help measure. Because it requires no special equipment apart from a clean pair of hands, it is a very portable therapy and an effective form of first aid.

In pregnancy and labour, acupressure has been shown to be very effective in helping to relieve different types of pain and discomfort. Scientific studies have shown that gentle pressure on the tsubos stimulates the body to release endorphins, a group of amino acids produced by the pituitary gland. When released into the blood stream, endorphins have the effect of numbing the receptors in the central nervous system, suppressing pain and inducing an overall sense of calm, relaxation and well-being.

Acupressure is not really a diagnostic tool, although to some extent your practitioner will be able to 'feel' where there is an imbalance in your body. Most people consult an acupressure therapist to deal with existing problems such as backache.

It has proved very successful at relieving the nausea associated with early pregnancy and labour. The simple application of pressure on the pericardium 6, or P6 point (located two thumb-widths above the most prominent crease on the underside of the wrist) is very helpful for some, though not all, women. Stimulation of this point, however, is less likely to relieve nausea which is accompanied by vomiting. You can apply pressure to the P6 point with your thumb or with a special wrist band which is available from the chemist.

Acupressure is also useful for relieving headaches, neck and upper back stiffness, lower back pain and, of course, labour pains. Contact the Shiatsu Society for a list of registered practitioners in your area.

WHAT TO EXPECT

Your therapist will want to know a little about your medical history, and you should in particular tell him or her of any medications you are taking. History-taking in acupressure is not as important as it is in many other alternative therapies. Nevertheless, your practitioner should always take the time to listen to what is ailing you.

Treatment usually takes place on the floor. You may be asked to lie on a futon, a thin mattress or simply on a folded blanket or towel. Some points on your body will feel more tender than others. This is usually a sign of imbalance. Gentle initial massage will help relieve that tender feeling. An acupressure session will usually last half an hour to an hour and you should be given a short time to rest and allow your body to integrate the subtle changes in its energy after each session.

Because acupressure is a gentle therapy, it is rare to have any negative reactions to it. Although most people leave the treatment room feeling relaxed, occasionally some may experience a less pleasant reaction. If you have been suffering from a chronic condition or if energy has been stagnant in a particular area of your body, moving that energy may release accumulated toxins into the body. As your body tries to rid itself of these toxins, you may experience a wide range of physical symptoms such as headaches or skin rashes, as well as emotional ones such as melancholy and fatigue. These symptoms should not last more than a few days. If you are at all worried by your reaction, always check with your practitioner.

TAKE CARE

Acupressure should not be applied in the following states:

• at a place on the body where there is an open wound, infection or swelling
• on any area of the skin which is red, inflamed or broken or where there is scar tissue, rash, blisters or varicose veins
• over the site of a broken bone or injured nerve or organ
• during pregnancy, the abdomen.

To avoid the risk of premature labour, acupressure should not be applied to the following sites in a woman who is less than 38 weeks' pregnant:

- small toe, including the toenail
- the back or inside of the lower legs, beginning at the knees
- the web of tissue between the thumb and forefinger, often referred to as the Hoku.

CHAPTER 20

YOGA AND ALEXANDER TECHNIQUE

───────── **WHAT IT'S BEST FOR** ─────────

FLEXIBILITY

POSTURE

VITALITY

RELAXATION

DIGESTIVE FUNCTION

HORMONAL FUNCTION

IMPROVING FOCUS AND CONCENTRATION

INTEGRATION OF BODY AND MIND

ELIMINATION OF WASTE AND TOXINS

MUSCLE TONE

CIRCULATION

☑ **Requires professional instruction**
☑ **Suitable for self-treatment after instruction**

Imagine feeling a sense of balance and harmony as you move through your day …

This is just one of the many benefits of practising the ancient art of yoga or the more recently developed Alexander Technique. The popularity of both these systems has increased in recent years as a way of maintaining a state of physical and emotional balance. More than any other form of bodywork or exercise regime, pregnant women may find that yoga and Alexander Technique combine a significant number of beneficial elements which support them through this time of transition.

To call these methods 'exercise', however, is somewhat misleading since both stem from philosophies which take a holistic view of health and well-being. In common with osteopathy and chiropractic, both yoga and Alexander Technique believe in the importance of the spine in relation to our health. Maintaining a strong, supple spine is seen as one way to promote good general health.

Being at your physical best during pregnancy has many benefits. It will ensure that your pregnancy is as trouble-free as it can be and that you are able to cope with the rigours of labour. It can speed your recovery from birth and help you through the demanding early days of parenthood. However, the effect does not stop there because a sense of physical well-being has an impact on almost every area of your life, including your emotions, creative expression and your mind. Both yoga and Alexander Technique provide a gentle way to promote this kind of well-being.

YOGA

Developed over the centuries, yoga is a unique way to increase the body's supply of energy. Most leisure centres and gyms now include yoga as part of their regular routine and classes are often among the most popular on offer.

The term yoga has come to encompass many different styles and philosophies. However, in the West the form of yoga which we are most familiar with is known as Hatha yoga. Although yoga is largely thought of as having been developed by men for men, there is some evidence that in prehistoric cultures women may have used the postures which were later adopted by the Yogis. In recent times women have shown an unprecedented interest in yoga and their influence has revolutionized the approach adopted by some practitioners.

While some forms of yoga seek to master the body and control the breath, others seek to work with the body and with the breath to establish a state of harmony in the body. While some forms of yoga seek (or so it seems) to defy gravity and may use forceful movements to attain certain postures, others work with gravity, allowing the body to adapt gradually to the postures and feel a greater sense of connection with the Earth. It is the less forceful type of yoga which has been adopted for pre-natal use and which is most often taught to pregnant women.

Many physicians who would otherwise be sceptical about alternative therapies are often surprisingly passionate about the benefits of yoga. Such views are supported by a number of clinical studies confirming the benefits of regular yoga, which can include lowered blood pressure and relief from stress and anxiety, as well as from physical complaints such as arthritis and asthma.

In general, however, yoga is not used to create health or to cure disease. Instead its aim is to create an environment, internally and externally, in which the individual can come to his or her own state of dynamic balance. Good health is not static and how we feel physically and emotionally will vary from day to day. The practice of yoga reinforces the interdependence of body and mind, allowing the individual to meet these day-to-day basic changes with greater ease.

For many devotees, yoga becomes a philosophy that offers guidance and insight into every aspect of life – the spiritual, the mental and the physical. It provides instruction on how to live and interact with others and even what to eat; many serious practitioners, for instance, are strict vegetarians. However, if you wish to practise yoga during pregnancy there is no need to take on the whole lifestyle unless you want to. Yoga is equally satisfying as a form of physical therapy and you will still derive great benefit from regular practice at this simple level.

The practice of yoga includes postures, breathing practices, progressive, deep relaxation and sometimes meditation. The most immediate benefit you will find from yoga is relaxation. We live in an age of anxiety and during pregnancy some women find that their anxieties become greater. In day-to-day living, most of our tensions are pushed to the back of our minds, where they become a part of the great, shadowy unconscious. Because we keep them hidden, we often describe ourselves as becoming tired, depressed or anxious for 'no good reason'. Even if you cannot locate the cause of your stress, you will certainly quickly become aware of the effect it has on your body, such as insomnia, poor digestion, headaches and lack of basic vitality. Through the practice of yoga you may find new insights into your problems and a gradual release of anxiety and tension.

Postures

The body postures, known as *asanas*, involve stretching movements which help strengthen, tone and balance the body and mind. They were originally used by the Indian philosophers to improve physical stamina and postural alignment, enabling them to sit in a balanced and still way for long periods of meditation.

More recently we have begun to learn that the postures used in yoga can also rejuvenate the body at a very deep level. The way this is achieved is complex, but includes three basic beneficial actions:

• increasing circulation to the brain, spine and specific organs and glands while also providing a massaging and/or stimulating action on certain areas of the body
• deep breathing and visualizing specific areas of the body can help to send an extra supply of blood and oxygen to them
• the nerves from the spinal column branch out to all the organs and glands; by increasing the spine's flexibility, the postures ensure a healthy central nervous system with a good connection to all parts of the body.

Breathing

Many types of yoga use specially developed breathing techniques, known as *pranayamas*. During pregnancy these will be as useful, if not more so, than any prescribed breathing practice. The reason for this is that they encourage you to find your own rhythm instead of following someone else's programme. Since the rhythm of your labour will be individual to you, it is important to connect with this idea and work on finding a breathing pattern which is uniquely relaxing to you.

There are two main uses of breathing practices in yoga:

• aligning the movement into and out of the postures with breathing; so, for example, some movements are done with the out-breath and others on an in-breath
• *pranayama* is both cleansing and revitalizing; often it involves specific breathing practices which encompass more than just breathing in and out, and include the ideas of life force, energy and vitality.

The Western way of breathing is often shallow and grasps sharply at the in-breath. In yoga, breathing practices help the breathing to be slower and more rhythmic. Some teachers emphasize the importance of the out-breath, maintaining that a full out-breath will improve the circulation of various bodily fluids, increase energy and enable wastes and toxins to be removed more easily.

Focused Awareness and Relaxation

Most yoga sessions include a period of relaxation with focused awareness or meditation, usually at the beginning or end of each session. Some people use this time to get in touch with themselves or their babies, others focus on affirmations or visualizations.

The reflective aspect of yoga is important, since the *asanas* and *pranayamas* also involve focused attention and work on the mind as well as the physical body. This is particularly helpful in this computer and video age, where we are all used to assimilating things quickly and on a superficial level, so that the spiritual 'muscle' of concentration has become very flabby.

Some antenatal yoga classes will have a period of reflection about your body, your baby and the coming birth. This is a good time to monitor your emotions and the way your body responds when you give your full attention to these things. When you visualize your labour, for instance, does your heart start to pump? Does your mouth go dry? Even if you appear calm on the outside, your body may be telling you that your anxiety needs more attention.

In more advanced yoga sessions there may also be a period of meditation. In the yogic sense, meditation is different from contemplation or visualization. Meditation in yoga involves sitting in an upright, still posture and clearing the mind of activity by focusing on one simple object. The object for meditation can be a simple image, a sound (sometimes called a *mantra*) or the natural rhythm of the breath. It can be quite a challenge to be quiet and still when our lives are so full of constant stimulation, but it can also be a relief and a welcome respite. The process of meditation, in which we continually let go of any thoughts that arrive, brings us closer to being centred and peaceful.

YOGA IN PREGNANCY

Yoga can claim good results with a number of physical problems in pregnancy. Chief among these are constipation, nausea, heartburn, mood swings, fluid retention and related complications such as Carpal Tunnel Syndrome and varicosities.

Many women, however, first approach their yoga teacher because they would like to find a gentle way of relaxing during pregnancy. Yoga can help the pregnant woman to consciously relax and can support her in her need to be more inward-looking. Because yoga is generally practised in a quiet atmosphere where the woman is encouraged to let all her other concerns pass away, it can help the mother get in touch with herself and her own needs as well as keeping in touch with her developing baby.

In this relaxed state the body can begin to repair itself. Your heart rate will slow, your breathing will become more efficient at releasing toxins from the body and your blood sugar levels will even out. If you are very busy or have a very stressful life, it is particularly important that you give your body a regular opportunity to repair some of the damage caused by stress.

Active Birth teachers use yoga as a major part of their antenatal preparation. However, pre-natal yoga classes are now springing up all over the country. Even if you are experienced at yoga, it might still be a good idea to go to a class to review which postures are suitable and which ones are not for pregnancy. If you are new to yoga, instruction is essential. Choose the teacher and group you feel most comfortable with, since the atmosphere in which you practise yoga enhances its effect.

YOGA IN LABOUR

There are no specific postures for use in labour. However, if you have been taking yoga classes throughout pregnancy you will be armed with many skills to help you give birth. Several yoga postures can be adapted in various stages of labour. Thus a woman may find that sitting in the tailor posture helps her to focus on her breathing in early labour, or taking up a position similar to the cat posture helps to ease the pain of a backache labour. The way you have learned to listen to and work with your body and your breathing and with gravity, as well as your improved

The Tailor Posture

This posture benefits the whole pelvic area, increasing circulation and mobility of the joints. It also helps to improve posture, relax the pelvic floor muscles and widen the pelvic dimensions in preparation for birth.

1 Sit comfortably on the floor with your feet in front of you (you can sit with your back against a wall if it is more comfortable).

2 Bring the soles of your feet together and draw them close to your body. The outside edges of your feet should be touching and the soles of the feet opening towards the ceiling. You can place a cushion under your thighs for support if you need to.

Note: Never force or strain in this position. If your feet won't come close to your body or your thighs do not touch the ground don't worry. Go as far as you comfortably can. With practice you will become more supple and reap more benefits. This posture should not be practised by women with Symphysis Pubic Disorder.

The Cat Posture

This posture can relieve the pressure of the fetus on the nerves and blood vessels of the lower pelvis and upper thighs. It also relieves backache and improves spinal flexibility and can strengthen the spine.

1 Kneel squarely on all fours with your hands directly beneath your shoulders and your body and head parallel to the floor. Inhale and slowly drop your back. Then spread your buttocks and raise your head and neck, keeping the face relaxed throughout.

2 As you exhale tuck your pelvis under, arch the spine and lower your head. Repeat several times, alternating a concave spine with a curled-up one.

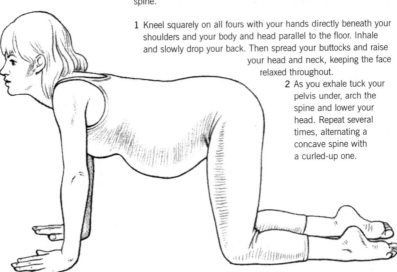

ability to focus, will all combine to help you cope more confidently with the demands of labour.

Because it promotes flexibility and strength, yoga will also help you to move more naturally and with greater ease during contractions. This, in turn, will help your labour progress more smoothly and make it less tiring.

WHAT TO EXPECT

Your yoga class will last between one and two hours and will usually involve a small group of 5 to 15 people. Teachers vary according to what they expect you to bring; many already have special yoga mats and occasionally belts available for their students, whereas some require you to bring your own. It is important that you wear loose, comfortable clothing to encourage freedom of movement. Socks are better than tights since they can be removed to give you more stability during standing postures.

Yoga sessions usually involve warming-up exercises at the beginning and a period of relaxation at the end. In between, your instructor will usually provide a varied programme of standing and floor postures and breathing exercises which you can also practise at home.

Make sure that you tell your teacher that you are pregnant, how far along you are and whether you have any pregnancy-related conditions such as pelvic pain or blood-pressure fluctuations. This information is important since there are certain postures which are not appropriate during pregnancy.

You should not feel any strain or pain in any of the postures you do. If you do, or if you begin to feel lightheaded or uncomfortable in any way, come out of the posture. Yoga is not a competition – though in a very few classes it can feel that way. You are not there to see how much longer you can hold a posture or how much more flexible you can be than the woman on the mat next to you. The only person you are doing it for is yourself. Know your limits and respect them.

You can find qualified yoga teachers through the British Wheel of Yoga and the Scottish Yoga Teachers' Association (*see* page 303).

TAKE CARE

Many women take up yoga for the first time in pregnancy. It is not advisable, however, to begin a yoga programme on your own if you have never practised it before or if you are expecting your first baby. To make sure that you get the most benefit out of the experience, always go to a class which is specially designed for pregnant women. There are many different schools of yoga and many different approaches. Not all of them, however (such as the new 'power yoga') are suitable for pregnant women.

Your ligaments will be much softer during pregnancy and you may be surprised by how easy some of the postures seem. However, softened ligaments also mean that it is much easier to push yourself too far and end up damaging your back or pelvis. During pregnancy, err on the side of caution and don't force your legs wide apart, either in standing or sitting postures. This is particularly important for women with symphysis pubis dysfunction (a painful condition, exacerbated by pregnancy, which makes any weight-bearing movement excruciating). If you are suffering from low blood pressure, postures which involve standing motionless for extended periods of time can make the condition worse.

While there are many excellent books on the subject of yoga, these should not be used as a substitute for classes, especially during pregnancy.

ALEXANDER TECHNIQUE

This technique is often thought of as a simple mixture of breathing and posture, but these aspects are only a part of the Alexander Technique. Like yoga, it is a whole approach to life which can help an individual become more aware of themselves in an everyday context. Through Alexander Technique you quickly become aware of the enormous strain (for instance through poor posture, bending and sitting incorrectly) you may be putting your body under each day.

The founder of Alexander Technique was an actor, F. Matthias Alexander. During the early part of his career he would habitually lose his voice. In searching for the cause and the cure, he found that by improving his posture he could regain his voice. This became the starting point for an entire system which aims to re-educate the person on how to move naturally, with a minimum of strain, especially on the head, neck and back – areas which affect our functioning as a whole.

Alexander Technique can help you let go of tensions which you may have been holding in your body for months, even years. Simply sitting or standing in an unbalanced way will put certain muscles under continual stress. Learning to move in a different way can help to release those tensions and many people report a feeling of liberation as they begin to practise Alexander Technique. In helping the student to relearn natural movement, Alexander teachers can also claim success in relieving such problems as depression, back trouble, exhaustion, respiratory problems, headaches, hypertension and digestive disorders.

The modern view of the body is it must be kept in line, yet many physical therapies show us that, in fact, the body obeys, even colludes with, our innermost instructions. The problem is that we are often unaware of the instructions we are sending our bodies. Alexander Technique is a way of becoming aware of the way body and mind interact and of enabling more constructive choices in the way we use our bodies.

Alexander Technique does not use meditation, exercises or relaxation, nor does it attempt to exert control over the breath. Alexander believed that breathing was largely an automatic process and that when the whole self was in harmony, correct breathing came naturally. Alexander also disputed the value of simply 'doing exercise' to become healthy. He believed that if a person's body sense was faulty, for instance through years of poor posture, it would be as unreliable a guide in exercise as it was in daily activities. Without awareness of the way we hold ourselves, exercise may further disturb the head, neck and back relationship, reinforcing, rather than correcting, physical problems.

He also believed that just exercising to correct specific problems might simply shift the tension to some other area of the body. A good example of this is sit-ups. Even the gentler types, such as the curl-ups used to tone slack abdominal muscles, can be overdone, creating a strain in the neck or other new health problems. There is also the problem of the 'high' which some people feel after vigorous repetitive exercise such as aerobics. Often this chemical response to such exercise can mask high-impact damage to soft tissues and joints.

But perhaps Alexander's biggest objection to exercise is that we often approach it as if body and mind were separate. To use the example of the abdominal muscles again, women habitually contract their abdominal muscles in the belief that this action gives the appearance of a flatter stomach. But contraction of these muscles is also associated with emotional repression and loss of body awareness in the whole abdominal/pelvic area.

ALEXANDER TECHNIQUE IN PREGNANCY

With Alexander Technique, the way you move when performing everyday tasks such as bending, tying your shoes, walking up stairs, squatting, sitting, raising yourself from a sitting or lying position and picking objects up from the floor will become conscious. You will be shown a series of better ways to do all these things which, when incorporated into your day-to-day activities, will take the strain off specific areas of your body. In this process of unlearning, other physical complaints such as backache and headache often disappear.

In pregnancy, Alexander Technique can help you to accommodate the changes in yourself as your baby grows. For example, many women respond to the size of their growing baby, by adopting a swayback stance, which puts pressure on the lower (lumbar) spine. Through Alexander Technique, you can learn to carry the weight of your baby in a way that still allows your spine to be long and strong. This, in turn, helps you to walk more easily, rather than falling into an uneven waddle which may cause discomfort in the hips and pelvis.

Alexander Technique may also have a role to play in ensuring that your baby is in an optimal position to be born. The number of babies who are in unfavourable positions before labour – such as the breech or transverse lie, or the posterior position, where the baby's back is facing the mother's back – are on the rise. Improved posture and better sitting and resting habits can provide more room in the pelvis for the baby to turn.

Alexander Technique can also be valuable in helping with pregnancy-related problems such as shoulder and neck tension and pelvic pain, including symphysis pubis dysfunction and hip pain.

ALEXANDER TECHNIQUE IN LABOUR

Like yoga, everything you learn in the course of an Alexander Technique lesson will come into play during labour. Instead of becoming tense in response to pain you may feel more conscious of your body and better able to direct its movements in response to the pain of labour.

Many women who have taken Alexander lessons use movement on all fours, or 'monkey' type movements during labour. These ways of moving allow more spaciousness in the pelvic area, and so help the baby in its passage into the outside world. In both these types of movements, you bend at the hips, knees and ankles, allowing the spine to be long. This contrasts with the way we tend to bend forward in our culture, which often involves bending from the waist, putting pressure on the back and reducing the space in front for the woman and her baby. Your Alexander teacher will help you learn how to move in these ways so that you feel more used to them before labour. The same ways of moving will be invaluable to you in lifting and carrying your new baby.

Although Alexander Technique does not rely on specific breathing exercises, one way of breathing, called the 'whispered ah' has proved helpful in labour. This method of breathing in a relaxed way, in through the nose and out through the mouth with an 'ah' sound, can be quite useful during contractions. In doing this you may feel your throat muscles begin to release. Some practitioners believe that there is a direct connection between the neck muscles and those in the neck of the womb, or cervix. When one set of muscles is relaxed, the other is as well.

Perhaps the main benefit of Alexander lessons is that you will have unlearned the idea that your body is your enemy. (In fact, the opposite is sometimes true: we tend to be enemies to our own bodies.) This takes an enormous amount of fear out of the process of giving birth.

WHAT TO EXPECT

Alexander Technique is taught by teachers, not therapists; you will be a pupil, not a patient. Sessions usually last 45 minutes to an hour and instruction is usually on a one-to-one basis, although a very few teachers may occasionally run group sessions. Your teacher will be particularly interested in how you use your body and may wish to observe you doing certain everyday movements such as sitting and standing. Your teacher will then begin to re-educate you in the use of your body, encouraging more conscious thinking, awareness and the minimum of effort. This is done by helping you to recognize habitual patterns of reaction and movement, leading you to a new, more constructive organization of your self, mind and body together.

Some of these more 'natural' positions may not feel quite natural at first, but the more you practise the more you will feel tensions in your body ebbing away.

Almost every session with your teacher will include some time lying on your back with knees raised and your head raised slightly. Usually some form of support, such as two or three books, is used. This position allows the release of tension through the whole body. Lying in this way for 20 minutes each day during early pregnancy is very relaxing, but in later pregnancy, resting on your side or leaning over a birth ball is usually more comfortable and ensures continued blood supply to your baby.

Your Alexander teacher will also give you some techniques for maintaining ease of movement in pregnancy and beyond and some provide postnatal classes. After around 30 sessions you should be able to continue practising Alexander Technique on your own.

The Society of Teachers of the Alexander Technique and Alexander Technique International (*see* page 302) can help you find a teacher in your area.

PART III
FINDING OUT MORE

YOUR BIRTH PLAN

Writing a birth plan serves as a statement to your carers and it also serves a purpose for you. It is a consciousness-raising exercise which helps you to prioritize and provides a structure within which you can sort through the complexities of modern maternity care. It forces you to go beneath the surface 'shoulds' and 'oughts' to the nitty-gritty of what you want out of your individual experience of pregnancy and birth. When a woman approaches the task of pregnancy and birth with this level of consciousness she is already halfway to a satisfying birth experience.

This book suggests many kinds of alternatives to the common experience of pregnancy and birth. Not all of them will necessarily be right for you. Whatever your view of birth, your birth plan should be written to express what is most important to you about pregnancy and labour. You should be able to say what pregnancy and birth mean to you and your partner. You should feel free to express your beliefs and values. You should also aim to include practical information along the following lines:

- Your chosen place for the birth.
- Your choice of birth partner(s), whether you would like your other children to be present (usually only possible at home births).
- Which antenatal procedures you wish to have or avoid, such as ultrasound, the use of a Doppler to listen to the baby's heart, and what alternatives, if any, such as Pinard or stethoscope, you propose.
- Which routine procedures in labour you wish to have or avoid, such as rupture of the membranes, fetal monitoring, induction and any alternatives you may choose.
- How you would like your birth to be, in other words whether you would like to be mobile during labour, to eat and drink when you need to, what position(s) you would like to try and give birth in, whether you

wish to have an unhurried second stage, whether you wish to labour and/or give birth in water, etc.

• How you feel about pain relief and what alternatives to conventional drugs you might wish to use.

• How you would like the third stage of your labour to go, i.e. do you want to deliver your placenta naturally and wait until the umbilical cord stops pulsating before it is cut? Or do you want to have an injection of syntometrine, in which case the cord must be cut beforehand?

• Whether you are willing to be attended by students antenatally and/or in labour.

• Whether you wish to hold and/or nurse your baby immediately after delivery and whether you wish to have some time alone with your baby and your partner after the birth.

• A request that any 'emergency' interventions are explained to you fully and your consent sought before they are implemented.

• Whether you agree to vitamin K being administered to your baby after birth and, if so whether it will it be by mouth or intramuscular injection.

• Your decision to breastfeed and, if so, instructions not to give your baby water or supplemental feeds while in hospital.

• You may also want to consider what you would do if for any reason your baby needs to be taken into special care, i.e. will you breastfeed.

Of course, you do not have to make a birth plan at all. But if you can't face writing it all down it is a good idea for you and your partner to think about and talk about all of the elements mentioned above. The information in the preceding chapters should help you to clarify your thoughts.

The single most important point about birth plans is this: *don't paint yourself into a corner with them.* Leave yourself room to respond to the way that your individual pregnancy and labour progresses. It's easy to fall into the trap of believing that once you have made a birth plan you must stick to it no matter what. This is not the case and, in fact, the word 'plan' is very misleading.

No one can plan for birth, not a GP, a midwife, an obstetrician or a mother. Your baby might surprise you by turning into an awkward position or taking longer to come than you expected (very common with first births). You may decide during labour that you wish to use some form of pain relief, but because you've written down in your 'plan' that you didn't want any, you are left with feelings of having 'failed' in some way. Early in your pregnancy you may have envisaged your labour as a kind of ongoing party with your partner, your best friend and half a dozen of your closest relatives by your side. But as time passes you may want something more private and will need to be able to change your mind with a clear conscience.

Think instead of a birth guideline and give yourself permission to deviate from the 'plan' or change your mind completely in order that you may respond appropriately to your and your baby's individual needs during pregnancy and labour.

Appendix 2 Essential Nutrients

Vitamin	Function	Best natural source
Vitamin A	Antioxidant and immune system booster. Essential for night vision. Promotes healthy skin, keeps outer layers of tissue and organs healthy.	Fish liver oil, liver, green and yellow vegetables, eggs, milk and dairy, yellow fruits.
B1 (Thiamine)	Aids digestion and is essential for energy production. Keeps nervous system, muscles and heart functioning normally.	Yeast, rice husks, wholewheat, oatmeal, peanuts, pork, most vegetables, bananas, milk.
B2 (Riboflavin)	Aids the metabolism of carbohydrates, fats and proteins. Necessary to repair and maintain healthy skin, nails and hair. Helps regulate body acidity.	Milk, liver, kidney, yeast, cheese, leafy green vegetables, fish, eggs.
B3 (Niacin)	Essential for energy production and brain function. Helps balance blood sugar and cholesterol levels. Promotes healthy skin. Can help prevent headaches.	Liver, mushrooms, tuna, chicken, salmon, lamb, asparagus, cabbage, tomatoes, mackerel, turkey, courgettes and squash, cauliflower, whole wheat products, brewer's yeast, kidney, wheat germ, fish, eggs, roasted peanuts, avocados, dates, figs, prunes.
B5 (Pantothenic Acid)	Essential for brain and nerves. Aids energy production and fat metabolism. Combats stress. Maintains healthy skin and hair.	Meat, wholegrains, wheat germ, bran, kidney, liver, heart, green vegetables, brewer's yeast, nuts, chicken, molasses.
B6 (Pyridoxine)	Aids digestion, brain function and hormone production. Helps balance sex hormones. Natural anti-depressant and diuretic. Alleviates nausea and muscle cramps.	Watercress, bananas, squash, broccoli, cauliflower, asparagus, lentils, red kidney beans, onions, brewer's yeast, wheat bran, wheat germ, liver, kidney, heart, cantaloupe, cabbage, molasses, milk, eggs, beef, seeds, nuts.
B12 (cyanocobalamin)	Helps the body utilize proteins. Necessary for energy production. Helps prevent anaemia. Improves concentration, memory and balance. Combats stress.	Oysters, sardines, lamb, shrimp, cottage cheese, poultry, cheese, liver, beef, pork, eggs, milk, kidney.
Biotin	Helps the body use essential fats. Promotes healthy skin, hair and nerves. Eases muscle pains.	Peas, tomatoes, cauliflower, lettuce, grapefruit, watermelon, sweetcorn, almonds, fruits, brewer's yeast, beef, liver, eggs, milk, kidney, unpolished rice.
Folic Acid (folacin)	Essential for brain and nerve function. Taken preconceptually and in early pregnancy, can help prevent neural tube defects. Helps prevent anaemia and can protect against intestinal parasites and food poisoning.	Dark green leafy vegetables, carrots, yeast, peanuts, sesame seeds, hazelnuts, walnuts, liver, egg yolk, melons, apricots, pumpkin, avocado, beans, whole wheat and dark rye flour.
Vitamin C (ascorbic acid)	Antioxidant and immune system booster. Fights stress. Heals wounds, A natural laxative. Improves elasticity of the skin.	Citrus fruits, peppers, watercress, berries, lemons, kiwi, melon, green and leafy vegetables, tomatoes, cauliflower, potato and sweet potato.
Vitamin D (ergocalciferol, cholecalciferol)	Helps the body utilize calcium and maintain strong bones. Can help in the treatment of conjunctivitis. Taken with A and C can boost immune system function.	Oily fish such as herring, mackerel, salmon and sardines, milk, cottage cheese, oysters, eggs.
Vitamin E (d-alpha tocopherol)	Antioxidant. Helps the body use oxygen. Keeps heart and circulatory system healthy. Improves skin and hastens wound healing. Aids fertility. Alleviates fatigue.	Unrefined sunflower and corn oils, wheat germ, soya beans, salmon, sardines, tuna, peanuts, broccoli, Brussels sprouts, sweet potatoes, leafy green vegetables, seeds, pulses, enriched flour, wholewheat, whole grain cereals, eggs.

	Function	Best natural source
EFAs (essential fatty acids: omega 3 and omega 6	Necessary for brain and nerve function. Has a role in preventing pre-eclampsia. Lowers cholesterol. Improves heart function.	Vegetable oils (wheat germ, linseed, sunflower, safflower, soya and peanut) peanuts, sunflower seeds, pumpkin seeds, hemp seeds, sesame seeds, walnuts, pecans, almonds, avocados, oily fish.
Vitamin K (phylloquinone)	Controls blood clotting.	Leafy green vegetables, potatoes, watercress, peas, beans, yoghurt, alfalfa, egg yolk, sunflower oil, soyabean oil, fish liver oils, kelp.
Mineral	**Function**	**Best natural source**
Calcium	Necessary for a healthy heart, nerves and muscles. Improves skin, bone and teeth. Can relieve aching muscles and reduce cramping. Maintains the acid–alkaline balance of the body.	Milk and milk products, all cheeses, brewer's yeast, prunes, corn tortillas, parsley, soyabeans, sardines, salmon, peanuts, walnuts, sunflower seeds, dried beans, green vegetables.
Chromium	Balances blood sugar levels, normalizes hunger and reduces cravings. Essential for a healthy heart.	Brewer's yeast, wholemeal and rye bread, green peppers, parsnips, cornmeal, lamb, potatoes, oysters, eggs, chicken, corn oil, clams.
Iron	Prevents anaemia and fatigue. Improves skin tone. Promotes resistance to disease and aids wound healing.	Pork liver, beef kidney, heart and liver, farina, raw clams, dried peaches, red meat, egg yolk, oysters, nuts and seeds, raisins, beans, asparagus, molasses, oatmeal.
Magnesium	Essential for energy production. Strengthens bones and teeth. Promotes healthy muscles including the heart muscle and in pregnancy the uterus. Maintains a healthy nervous system.	Nuts, dates and figs, lemons, grapefruit, yellow corn, seeds, dark-green vegetables, apples.
Manganese	Necessary for healthy bones, cartilage, tissue and nerves. Helps alleviate fatigue. Stabilizes blood sugar. Required for proper brain function.	Grapes, nuts, watercress, pineapple, okra, endive, celery, berries, lima beans, beetroot, green leafy vegetables, peas, egg yolks, whole grain cereals.
Molybdenum	Helps the body eliminate waste products. Helps prevent anaemia. Strengthens teeth.	Tomatoes, wheat germ, pork, lentils, beans, dark-green leafy vegetables, whole grains.
Phosphorus	Builds muscle tissue. Aids lactation. Maintains bones and teeth. Aids energy production and metabolism.	Present in most foods.
Potassium	Helps in the elimination of waste products. Maintains the body's fluid balance. Promotes healthy nerves and muscles. Involved in metabolism and maintaining blood sugar levels.	Citrus fruits, watercress, all green leafy vegetables, mint leaves, sunflower seeds, bananas, potatoes, mushrooms, cauliflower, pumpkin, courgettes.
Selenium	Antioxidant. Reduces inflammation. Promotes healthy heart. Needed for metabolism.	Tuna, oysters, molasses, cottage cheese, mushrooms, herring, wheat germ, bran, onions, tomatoes, broccoli, courgette.
Sodium	Maintains the body's water balance. Necessary for nerve and muscle function.	Salt, olives, shrimp, miso, celery, beetroot, crab, ham and bacon, shellfish, carrots, beets, artichokes, dried beef, brains, kidney.
Zinc	Important for healing, essential for growth. Controls hormones which are messengers from the reproductive organs. Relieves stress. Aids bone and teeth formation. Essential for energy production. Boosts immunity.	Ginger root, beef, lamb, pork, wheat germ, brewer's yeast, shrimp, pumpkin seeds, nuts, eggs, turnips, oats, dry split peas, ground mustard.

BIBLIOGRAPHY

General

Complementary Therapies for Pregnancy and Childbirth, Denise Tiran and Sue Mack, London: Bailliere Tindall, 1995

Encyclopaedia of Natural Medicine, Michael Murray and Joseph Pizzorno, London: Optima, 1995

The Handbook of Complementary Medicine, Stephen Fulder, London: Century, 1989

Your Body Speaks Your Mind, Debbie Shapiro, London: Piatkus, 1996

Alternatives in Healing, Simon Mills and Steven J. Finando, New York: Plume, 1988

Natural Healing for Women, Susan Curtis and Romy Frasier, London: Pandora, 1991

Alternative Healthcare for Women, Patsy Westcott, London: Grapevine, 1987

Natural Healthcare for Women, Belinda Grant Viagas, Dublin: New Leaf, 1997

Pregnancy and Birth

Pregnant Feelings, Rahima Baldwin and Terra Palmarini, Berkeley, Cailfornia: Celestial Arts, 1986

Transformation Through Pregnancy, Claudia Panuthos, Massachusettes: Bergin & Garvey, 1984

Planning for a Healthy Baby, Belinda Barnes and Suzanne Gail Bradley, London: Ebury, 1990

Entering the World, Michel Odent, London: Penguin, 1984

Every Woman's Birth Rights, Pat Thomas, London: Thorsons, 1996

Every Birth is Different, Pat Thomas, London: Headline, 1997

Pregnancy: The Common Sense Approach, Pat Thomas, Dublin: New Leaf, 1999

Your Natural Pregnancy, Anne Charlish, London: Boxtree, 1995

Spiritual Midwifery, Ina May Gaskin, Saummertown, Tennessee: The Book Publishing Co, 1990

The New Active Birth, Janet Balaskas, London: Thorsons, 1991

The Active Birth Partners Handbook, Janet Balaskas, London: Sidgwick & Jackson, 1986

Natural Pregnancy, Janet Balaskas, London: Gaia, 1999

The New Pregnancy & Childbirth, Sheila Kitzinger, London: Dorling Kindersley, 1997

The Experience of Childbirth, Sheila Kitzinger, London: Penguin, 1987

Ourselves as Mothers, Sheila Kitzinger, London: Bantam Press, 1992

Trust Your Body! Trust Your Baby, Andrea Frank Henkart, London: Bergin & Garvey, 1995

Birth Traditions and Modern Pregnancy, Jacqueline Vincent Pirya, Shaftesbury: Element, 1992

Eve's Wisdom, Deborah Jackson, London: Duncan Baird, 1999

Three in a Bed, Deborah Jackson, London: Bloomsbury, 1990

Alternative Maternity, Nicky Wesson, London: Optima, 1989

The Encyclopedia of Pregnancy and Birth, Janet Balaskas and Yehudi Gordon, London: Little Brown, 1992

Research and Information

A Guide to Effective Care in Pregnancy and Childbirth, Murray Enkin et al, Oxford: Oxford University Press, 1995

Understanding Diagnostic Tests in the Childbearing Year, Anne Frye, Portland, Oregon: Labrys Press, 1997

Caesarean Birth in Britain, Colin Francombe et al, London: Middlesex University Press/NCT, 1993

Obstetric Myths and Research Realities, Henci Goer, London: Bergin & Garvey, 1995

Where to Be Born – The Debate and the Evidence, Alison Macfarlane and Rhona Campbell, Oxford: National Perinatal Epidemiological Unit, 1994

Safer Childbirth? – A Critical History of Maternity Care, Marjorie Tew, London: Routledge, 1995

Pursuing the Birth Machine – The Search for Appropriate Birth Technology, Marsden Wagner, NSW, Australia: ACE Graphics, 1994

Waterbirth Unplugged, Beverley Lawrence Beech (ed), Hale Cheshire: Books For Midwives, 1994

The Secret Life of the Unborn Child, Dr Thomas Verny and John Kelly, London: Sphere, 1982

Beginning Life, Geraldine Lux Flanagan, London: Dorling Kindersley, 1996

Pain in Childbearing and its Control, Rosemary Mander, London: Blackwell Science, 1998

Acupuncture

The Web that Has no Weaver, Ted J. Kaptchuk, London: Rider, 1986

Aromatherapy

The Fragrant Pharmacy, Valerie Ann Worwood, London: Bantam, 1998

Aroma Science – The Chemistry & Bioactivity of Essential Oils, Dr Maria Lis-Balchin, East Horsley, Surrey: Amberwood, 1995

The Art of Aromatherapy, Robert Tisserand, Saffron Walden: Daniel, 1989

Shirley Price's Aromatherapy Workbook, Shirley Price, London: Thorsons, 1993

Principles of Aromatherapy, Cathy Hopkins, London: Thorsons, 1996

Herbs & Flower Remedies

The New Holistic Herbal, David Hoffman, Shaftesbury: Element: 1990

Wise Woman Herbal for the Childbearing Year, Susan S. Weed, Woodstock, New York: Ash Tree, 1986

Herbal Remedies for Women, Amanda McQuade Crawford,

The Women's Guide to Herbal Medicine, Carol Rogers, London: Hamish Hamilton, 1995

The Complete Floral Healer, Ane McIntyre, London: Gaia, 1996

Holistic Herbal for Mother and Baby, Kitty Campion, London: Bloomsbury, 1996

Flower Remedies, Peter Mansfield, London: Vermilion, 1997

Flower Remedies for Women, Christine Wildwood, London: Thorsons, 1994

Illustrated Handbook of the Bach Flower Remedies, Philip M. Chancellor, Saffron Walden: Daniel, 1986

The Scientific Validation of Herbal Medicine, Daniel B. Mowrey, New Canaan, Connecticut: Keats, 1986

Homeopathy
A Woman's Guide to Homeopathy, Dr Andrew Lockie and Dr Nicola Geddes, London: Hamish Hamilton, 1993
Everybody's Guide to Homeopathic Medicines, Stephen Cummings and Dana Ullman, London: Gollancz, 1986
Practical Homeopathy, Beth MacEoin, London: Bloomsbury, 1997
A Woman's Guide to Homeopathic Medicine, Dr Trevor Smith, Welingborough: Thorsons, 1985

Hypnotherapy
Principles of Hypnotherapy, Vera Peiffer, London: Thorsons, 1991
Hypnosis and Hypnotherapy, Hellmut W. A. Karle, London: Thorsons, 1988

Massage
The Book of Massage, Lucinda Liddell, London: Ebury Press, 1989

Nutrition
Food and Healing, Annemarie Colbin, New York: Ballantine, 1996
The Better Pregnancy Diet, Patrick Holford, London: ION Press, 1992
Healing Through Nutrition, Dr Melvyn R. Werbach, London: Thorsons, 1993
Nutritional Medicine, Dr Stephen Davies and Dr Alan Stewart, London: Pan, 1987
Shaping Up With Vitamins, Earl Mindell, London: Arlington, 1985
Healing Foods for Common Ailments, Dr Penny Stanway, London: Gaia, 1989
Aromatherapy in Your Diet, Daniele Ryman, London: Piatkus, 1996
Healthy Eating for You and Your Baby, Fiona Ford, Robert Fraser and Hilary Dimond, London: Pan, 1994

Principles of Nutritional Therapy, Linda Lazarides, London: Thorsons, 1996

GM Free, Sue Dibb and Tim Lobstein, London: Virgin, 1999

Osteopathy

Wilbur Cole, in J. M. Hoag, W. V. Cole and S. G. Brandford, *Osteopathic Medicine*, St Louis/New York: McGraw Hill, 1969

Dynamic Chiropractic Today, Michael Copland-Griffiths, London: Thorsons, 1991

Psychotherapy and Counselling

Understanding Ourselves, Joan Woodward, London: Macmillan, 1988

Psychology of Childbearing, Nora Tisdall, Hale, Cheshire: Books For Midwives, 1997

Songs From the Womb, Benig Mauger, Cork: The Collins Press, 1998

Reflexology

Reflexology – Foot Massage for Total Health, Inge Dougns and Suzzanne Ellis, Shaftesbury: Element, 1991

Shiatsu and Acupressure

Shiatsu for Women, Ray Ridolfi and Susanne Franzen, London: Thorsons, 1996

Acupressure for Common Ailments, Chris Jarmey and John Tindall, London: Gaia, 1991

Yoga

Preparing for Birth With Yoga, Janet Balaskas, Shaftesbury: Element, 1994

Yoga for Women, Paddy O'Brien, London: Thorsons, 1994

The Book of Yoga, Lucy Lidell and The Sivananda Yoga Centre, London: Ebury Press, 1995

Yoga for Everyone, Kareen Zebroff, London: Foulsham, 1995

The Alexander Technique – Natural Poise for Health, Richard Brennan, Shaftesbury: Element, 1991

WHO CAN HELP?

PREGNANCY AND BIRTH GENERAL

UK

Active Birth Centre
25 Bickerton Road
London N19 5JT
Tel: (0207) 561 9006
website address:
www/activebirthcentre.com

Association for Improvements in the Maternity Services (AIMS)
In England:
40 Kingswood Avenue
London NW6 6LS
Tel: (0208) 865 5585
website address: www.aims.org.uk

In Scotland:
40 Leamington Terrace
Edinburgh EH10 4JL
Tel: (0131) 229 6259

In Northern Ireland:
23 Station Mews
Todd's Hill
Saintfield
Co Down
Tel: (01238) 511786

British Association for Counselling
1 Regent Place
Rugby
Warwickshire CV21 2PJ
Tel: (01788) 550899/578328

Caesarean and VBCA Support
c/o Gina Lowdon
Park View, Mill Corner
North Warnborough
Hook, Hampshire RG29 1HB
Tel: (01256) 704871

Caesarean Support Network
c/o Sheila Tunstall
2 Hurst Park Drive
Huyton
Liverpool L36 1TF
Tel: (0151) 480 1184

Independent Midwives Association
94 Auckland Road
London SE19 2BD
Tel: (0208) 406 3172

Maternity Alliance
45 Beech Street
5th Floor
London EC2P 2LX
Tel: (0207) 588 8582

Midwives Information and Resource Service (MIDIRS)
9 Elmdale Road
Clifton
Bristol BS8 1SL
Tel: (0117) 925 1791

National Childbirth Trust (NCT)
Alexandra House
Oldham Terrace
London W3 6NH
Tel: (0208) 992 8637

US

Aromatherapy Market
PO Box 459
Newfield NY 14867
Tel: 607 546 7864

National Association of Childbearing
3123 Gottschall Road
Perkiomenville
PA 18074
Tel: 215 234 8068

La Leche League
1400 N Meacham Road
Schaumburg
IL 60173 4048
Tel: 847 519 7730

Lamaze International
1200 19th St NW
Suite 300
Washington DC 20036 2422
Tel: 800 368 4404

American College of Nurse Midwives
1522 K St NW 110
Washington DC 20005

Informed Homebirth
PO Box 3675
Ann Arbor
MI 48106
Tel: 313 662 6857

Australia

Australian Natural Therapists Association
PO Box 308
Melrose Park 5039
South Australia
Tel: 618 297 9533

OZ Child: Children Australia
PO Box 1310
South Melbourne
Victoria 3205
Tel: 03 9695 2211

Australian Traditional Medicine Society Limited
(Mailing)
PO Box 1027
Meadowbank
NSW 2114
(Office)
12/27 Bank Street
Meadowbank
NSW 2114

Childbirth Education Association of Australia (NSW) Limited
Suite 11
127 Forest Road
Hurstville 2220
Tel: 02 580 0399

The Childbirth Education Association (Brisbane) Inc
PO Box 208
Chermside 4032
Tel: 07 3359 9724

The Compassionate Friends
Bereaved Parents Support and
Information Centre
300 Camberwell Road
Camberwell
Victoria 3124
Tel: 03 9882 3355

**Relationships Australia
Queensland**
159 St Paul's Terrace
Brisbane
Queensland 4000
Tel: 07 3831 2005

Diabetes Australia
AVA House
5-7 Phipps Place
Deakin
ACT 2600
Tel: 616 285 3277

SPECIAL NEEDS

Alcoholics Anonymous (AA)
AA General Service Office
PO Box 1
Stonebow House
Stonebow
York YO1 2NJ
Tel: (01904) 644026

BLISS
17–21 Emerald Street
London WC1N 3QL
Tel: (0207) 831 9393

Narcotics Anonymous
PO Box 417
London SW10 0DP
Tel: (0207) 498 9005

**National Information for Parents
of Prematures – Education,
Resources and Support
(NIPPERS)**
28 Swyncombe Avenue
London W5
Tel: (0208) 847 4721

Pre-Eclampsia Society (PETS)
17 South Avenue
Holdbridge, Essex SS5 6HA
Tel: (01702) 232533

Quit
102 Gloucester Place
London W1H 3DA
Tel: (0207) 487 3000 (helpline –
phone between 9.30am and
5.30pm)

Relate: Marriage Guidance
Herbert Gray College
Little Church Street
Rugby CV21 3AP
Tel: (01788) 573241

Support after Termination for Fetal Abnormality (SAFTA)
29 Soho Square
London W1V 6JB
Tel: (0207) 439 6124

Stillbirth and Neonatal Death Society (SANDS)
28 Portland Place
London W1N 4DE
Tel: (0207) 436 5881

Twins and Multiple Births Association (TAMBA)
PO Box 30
Little Sutton
S. Wirral L66 1TH
Tel: (0151) 348 0020
Helpline:
Tel: (01732) 868000 7–11pm
weekdays; 10am–11pm weekends

POSTNATAL SUPPORT

Association of Breastfeeding Mothers
26 Herschell Close
London SE26 4TH
Tel: (0208) 778 4769

Avon Episiotomy Support Group
PO Box 130
Weston-super-Mare
Avon BS23 4YJ

CRY-SIS
BM CRY-SIS
London WC1N 3XX
Tel: (0207) 404 5011

Gingerbread
16–17 Clerkenwell Close
London EC2R 0AA
Tel: (0207) 336 8183
Northern Ireland: Tel: (01232) 231417
Scotland: Tel: (0141) 353 0953
Wales: Tel: (01792) 648728

La Leche League (Great Britain)
BM 3424
London WC1N 3XX
Tel: (0207) 242 1278
(24-hour answer-phone)

Meet-a-Mum Association (MAMA)
c/o Briony Hallam
58 Malden Avenue
South Norwood
London SE25 4HS
Tel: (0208) 656 7318

National Childminding
Association
c/o Veronica Day
8 Masons Hill
Bromley, Kent BR2 9EY

**United Kingdom Council for
Psychotherapy**
167–9 Great Portland Street
London W1N SF
Tel: (0207) 436 3002

ALTERNATIVE THERAPIES

UK

**Institute for Complementary
Medicine**
and
**The British Register of
Complementary Practitioners
(BRCP)**
PO Box 194
London SE16 1QZ
Tel: (0207) 237 5165

**British Complementary Medicine
Association (BCMA)**
249 Fosse Road
South Braunston
Leicester LE3 1AE
Tel: (0116) 282 5511

Shiatsu Society
Suite D
Barber House
Storey's Bar Road
Fengate
Peterborough
Cambs PE1 5YS
Tel: (01733) 758341

Association of Reflexologists
27 Old Gloucester Street
London WC1N 3XX
Tel: (0870 5773320)

**British Acupuncture Council
and Register**
63 Jeddo Road
London W12 9HQ
Tel: (0208) 735 0400

**British Medical Acupuncture
Society**
Newton House
Newton Lane
Whitley
Warrington
Cheshire WA4 4JA
Tel: (01925) 730727

Bach Flower Remedies
The Bach Centre
Mount Vernon
Sotwell
Wallingford
Oxfordshire OX10 9P2
Tel: (0491) 834678

Flower Essence Fellowship
Laura Farm Clinic
17 Carlincott
Peasedown St. John
Bath BA2 8AN

**Alexander Technique
International
(UK Region)**
66C Thurlestone Road
London SE27 0PD
Tel: (07071) 880253

**Society of Teachers of the
Alexander Technique (STAT)**
20 London House
266 Fulham Road
London SW10 0EL
Tel: (0207) 351 0828

**International Federation
of Aromatherapists**
2/4 Chiswick High Road
Stanford House
London W4 1TH
Tel: (0208) 742 2605

**International Society of
Professional Aromatherapists
(ISPA)**
ISPA House
82 Ashby Road
Hinckley
Leicestershire LE10 1SN
Tel: (01455) 637987

British Chiropractic Association
Blagrave House
Blagrave Street
Reading
Berkshire RG1 1QB
Tel: (0118) 950 5950

**British Society of Allergy,
Environmental and Nutritional
Medicine**
PO Box 7
Knighton
Powys LD7 1WT
(send SAE)

**National Institute of Medical
Herbalists**
56 Longbrook Street
Exeter EX4 6AH
Tel: (01392) 426022

**International Register of Consultant
Herbalists and Homeopaths**
32 King Edward Road
Swansea SA1 4LL
Tel: (01792) 655886

**British Homeopathic
Association**
27a Devonshire Street
London W1N 1RJ
Tel: (0207) 935 2163

Society of Homeopaths
2 Artizan Road
Northampton NN1 4HU
Tel: (01604) 621400

**British Hypnotherapy
Association**
67 Upper Berkley Street
London W1H 7DH
Tel: (0207) 723 4443

**British Association of
Nutritional Therapists**
BCM BANT
London
WC1N 3N1

Foresight
28 The Paddock
Godalming
Surrey GU7 1XD
Tel: (01483) 427839

**Society for Promotion of
Nutritional Therapy**
PO Box 47
Heathfield
East Sussex TN21 8ZX
Tel: (01435) 867007

**Institute for Optimum
Nutrition**
13 Blades Court
Deodar Road
London SW15 2NU
Tel: (0208) 877 9993

Soil Association
(organic food and farming
information)
86 Colston Street
Bristol BS1 5BB
Tel: (0117) 929 0661

**Women's Nutritional
Advisory Service (WNAS)**
PO Box 286
Lewes
East Sussex BN7 2QN

General Osteopathic Council
Osteopathy House
176 Tower Bridge Road
London SE1 3LU
Tel: (0207) 357 6655

**Centre for Stress
Management**
156 Westcombe Hill
Blackheath
London SE3 7DH
Tel: (0208) 293 4114

British Wheel of Yoga
BWY Central Office
1 Hamilton Place
Boston Road
Sleaford
Lincolnshire NG34 7ES
Tel: (01529) 306851

**Scottish Yoga Teachers'
Association**
268 Bath Street
Glasgow G2 4JR
Tel: (0141) 332 8507

US

Alliance/Foundation for Alternative Medicine
160 NW Widmer Place
Albany
OR 97321
Tel: 503 926 4678

American College of Advancement in Medicine
PO Box 3427
Laguna Hills
California 92654

American Counseling Association
5999 Stevenson Avenue
Alexandrea
Virginia
22304-9800

American Chiropractic Association
1701 Clarendon Boulevard
Arlington
Virginia 22209
Tel: 703 276 8800

American Herb Association
PO Box 1673
Nevada City
California 95959

American Holistic Medical Association
4101 Lake Boone Trail
Suite 201
Raleigh
NC 27607
Tel: 919 787 5181

American Holistic Nurses Association
PO Box 2130
2133 E Lakin Drive
Suite 2 Flagstaff
Arizona 86003-211130

Angelica's Traditional Herbs and Food
147 First Avenue, New York
NY 10003
Tel: 212 677 1549

The Aromatherapy Institute and Research
PO Box 1222
Fair Oaks
California 95628

American Academy of Osteopathy
3500 Depaw Boulevard
Suite 1080
Indianopolis
Indiana 46268 139
Tel: 317 879 1881

Association for Humanistic Psychology (International)
45 Franklin Street
315 San Francisco
CA 94102

Association of Bodyworkers and Massage Professionals
28677 Buffalo Park Road
Evergreen
Colorado 80439
Tel: 303 674 8478

Dr Edward Bach
Healing Society
644 Merrick Road Lynbrook
New York 11563
Tel: 516 825 2229

International Foundation
of Homeopathy
2366 Eastlake Avenue East
Ste 301
Seattle
WA 98102
Tel: 703 548 7790

International Association
of Yoga Therapists
109 Hillside Avenue
Mill Valley
California 94941
Tel: 415 383 4587

Nelson Bach USA Limited
Wilmington Technology Park
100 Research Drive
Wilmington
Massachusetts 01887-4406
Tel: 978 988 3833

Australia
Australian College of
Alternative Medicine
11 Howard Avenue
Mount Waverley
Victoria 3149

Australasian College of
Natural Therapies
620 Harris Street
Ultimo
NSW 2007
Tel: 02212 6699

Australian Traditional Medicine
Society
Suite 3, First Floor
120 Blaxland Road
Ryde
NSW 2112
Tel: 612 808 2825

The Australian Society of
Teachers of the Alexander
Technique
19 Princess Street
Kew
Victoria 3101
Tel: 0398 531 356

International Federation of
Aromatherapists
1/390 Burwood Road
Hawthorn
Victoria 3122
Tel: 03 9530 0067

Martin & Pleasance
Wholesale Pty Ltd
(Flower Essences)
PO Box 4
Collingwood
Victoria
NSW 3066
Tel: 419 9733

Australian College of
Oriental Medicine
24 Price Road
Lalorama
Victoria 3766

Australian Council on
Chiropractic and Osteopathic
Education
941 Nepean Highway
Mornington
Victoria 3931

National Herbalists
Association of Australia
Suite 305
BST House
3 Small Street
Broadway
NSW 2007
Tel: 02 211 6437

Australian Institute of
Homeopathy
7 Hampden Road
Artemon
Sydney
NSW 2064

Association of Massage
Therapists
18A Spit Road
Mosman
NSW 1088

Association of Reflexology
2 Stewart Avenue
Matraville
NSW 2036
Tel: 02311 2322

Australian College of Nutritional
and Environmental Medicine
13 Hilton Road
Beamaris
Victoria 3193
Tel: 03 9589 6088

International Yoga Teachers'
Association
c/o 14/15 Huddart Avenue
Normanhurst
NSW 2076

South Africa

**Western Cape SU Jok
Acupuncture Institute**
3 Periwinkle Close
Kommetjie 7975
Tel: 021 783 3460

SASTAT (Alexander Technique)
5 Leinster Road
Green Point 8001
Cape Town

Association of Aromatherapists
PO Box 23924
Claremont 7735
Tel: 021 531 297

The Herb Society of South Africa
PO Box 37721
Overport

**South African Naturopaths and
Herbalists Association**
PO Box 18663
Wynberg 7824

Inge Dougans (Reflexology)
PO Box 68283
Bryanston
Johannesburg 2021
Tel: 27 11 706 4206

INDEX

ABOUT THE AUTHOR

Pat Thomas writes widely in the field of alternative health for newspapers and magazines and has become a well-known and outspoken advocate of holistic, patient-centred care. She is the author of several highly acclaimed books, including *Every Woman's Birth Rights, Every Birth is Different* and *Pregnancy – The Common Sense Approach*, as well as several children's books. She is a contributing editor to the alternative health newsletter *Proof!* and, as a qualified psychotherapist and a birth counsellor, she is the alternative health adviser for *Pregnancy & Birth Magazine*. She is also an active member of AIMS (Association for Improvements in the Maternity Services) and Editor of their journal. Pat lectures widely and is a regular featured guest on TV and radio programmes throughout the UK. She lives in London with her son.